MW00592698

Atlas of Pediatrics in the Tropics
and Resource-Limited Settings

Editors

Jonathan M. Spector, MD, MPH, FAAP
Massachusetts General Hospital
Harvard Medical School
Harvard School of Public Health
Boston, MA

Timothy E. Gibson, MD, FAAP
UMASS Memorial Children's Medical Center
University of Massachusetts Medical School
Worcester, MA

Associate Editors

**Rana Chakraborty, MD, MSc,
FRCPCH, DPhil, FAAP**
Associate Professor of Pediatrics
Director, Ponce Family and Youth Clinic
Division of Infectious Diseases
Emory University School of Medicine
Atlanta, GA

Anna Mandalakas, MD, MS Epi, FAAP
Associate Professor of Pediatrics,
Global & Public Health
Case Western Reserve University
Cleveland, OH

Ben J. Marais, MD, PhD
Associate Professor of Pediatrics,
Health Sciences Faculty
Stellenbosch University
Tygerberg, South Africa

**Elizabeth Molyneux, MBBS, FRCP,
FRCPCH, FRCPCH(Hons), FCEM, OBE**
Professor of Paediatrics
University of Malawi
Blantyre, Malawi

**Alagiriswamy Parthasarathy, MBBS,
DCH, MD(Ped), FIAP**
Retired Senior Clinical Professor of
Pediatrics, Madras Medical College
Deputy Superintendent, Institute of Child
Health and Hospital for Children
Senior Consultant Pediatrician,
AP Child Care
Chennai, India

Javier Santisteban-Ponce, MD
Attending Physician, Department
of Pediatrics
Edgardo Rebagliati National
Hospital—EsSalud
Universidad Peruana Cayetano Heredia
Lima, Peru

American Academy of Pediatrics
DEDICATED TO THE HEALTH OF ALL CHILDREN™

American Academy of Pediatrics Department of Marketing and Publications

Maureen DeRosa, MPA, Director, Department of Marketing and Publications
Mark Grimes, Director, Division of Product Development
Martha Cook, Senior Product Development Editor
Carrie Peters, Editorial Assistant
Sandi King, MS, Director, Division of Publishing and Production Services
Theresa Wiener, Manager, Editorial Production
Kate Larson, Manager, Editorial Services
Peg Mulcahy, Manager, Graphic Design and Production
Jill Ferguson, Director, Division of Marketing
Linda Smessaert, Manager, Clinical and Professional Publications Marketing
Robert Herling, Director, Division of Sales

Library of Congress Control Number 2008941468
ISBN 978-1-58110-303-8
MA0447

The recommendations in this publication do not indicate an exclusive course of treatment or serve as a standard of care. Variations, taking into account individual circumstances, may be appropriate.

Brand names are furnished for identifying purposes only. No endorsement of the manufacturers or products listed is implied.

Every effort has been made to ensure that the drug selection and dosage set forth in this text are in accordance with the current recommendations and practice at the time of publication. It is the responsibility of the health care provider to check the package insert of each drug for any change in indications and dosage and for added warnings and precautions.

Printed in China

1 2 3 4 5 6 7 8 9 10

Suggested citation: Spector JM, Gibson TE. *Atlas of Pediatrics in the Tropics and Resource-Limited Settings*. Elk Grove Village, IL: American Academy of Pediatrics; 2009.

9-245/0509

*Dedicated to the children and their families
whose stories are described herein.*

Contributors

Bronwen J. Anders, MD, FAAP
Clinical Professor of Pediatrics
University of California, San Diego
San Diego, CA
Ancylostomiasis
Trichuriasis

Melanie Anspacher, MD
Pediatric Hospitalist, Children's National Medical Center
Assistant Professor of Pediatrics, The George Washington
   University Medical Center
Washington, DC
Melioidosis

Jorge Atouguia, MD, MSc, PhD
Associate Professor of Tropical Medicine, Department of
   Tropical Diseases
Instituto de Higiene e Medicina Tropical
Universidade Nova de Lisboa
Lisboa, Portugal
Trypanosomiasis, African

Komal Bajaj, MD, FAAP
Pediatric Hospitalist
Inova Fairfax Hospital for Children
Falls Church, VA
Hypothyroidism, Congenital

Bradley R. Berg, MD, PhD
President, Humanity for Children
Seattle, WA
Yaws

Francisco G. Bravo, MD
Associate Professor of Medicine and Pathology
Universidad Peruana Cayetano Heredia
Lima, Peru
Scabies

Judith Patricia Breña, MD
Research Associate
Instituto de Medicina Tropical Alexander von Humboldt
Universidad Peruana Cayetano Heredia
Lima, Peru
Toxocariasis

Frederick M. Burkle Jr, MD, MPH, FAAP, FACEP
Woodrow Wilson International Scholar
Senior Fellow, Harvard Humanitarian
    Initiative, Harvard University,
    Cambridge
Senior Associate Faculty, Department of
    International Health and Emergency
    Medicine, Johns Hopkins University
    Medical Institutions
Professor, Department of Community
    Emergency Health, Monash
    University Medical School
Melbourne, Australia
Plague
Scurvy

Mala Chhabra
Joint Director
National Institute of Communicable
    Diseases
New Delhi, India
Chikungunya Fever

Jean-Phillippe Chippaux, MD, DrSc
Directeur de Recherche
Mother's and Child's Health in
    Tropical Environment
Institut de Recherche pour le
    Développement
Paris, France
Snakebite

Scott J. Cohen, MD
Founder and Medical Director
Global Pediatric Alliance
Oakland, CA
Dengue
Giardiasis
Trachoma

Keri A. Cohn, MD, DTM&H
Fellow, Pediatric Infectious Diseases
    and Emergency Medicine
Children's Hospital Boston
Harvard Medical School
Boston, MA
Malnutrition
Viral Hemorrhagic Fever

Martine Debacker, MSc, MPH, PhD
Researcher, Mycobacteriology Unit
Institute of Tropical Medicine
Antwerpen, Belgium
Buruli Ulcer

Michael B. Dinerman, MD, FAAP
Emergency Medicine
Children's Healthcare of Atlanta
Piedmont Hospital
Atlanta, GA
Trypanosomiasis, American

Christiane Dolecek, MD
University of Oxford Clinical
    Research Unit
The Hospital of Tropical Diseases
Ho Chi Minh City, Vietnam
Typhoid Fever

Elizabeth M. Dufort, MD
Teaching Fellow in Pediatrics
Alpert Medical School of
    Brown University
Hasbro Children's Hospital/Rhode
    Island Hospital
Providence, RI
HIV and AIDS

Paul M. Emerson, PhD
Director, Trachoma Control Program
Codirector, Trachoma Control
    Program
The Carter Center
Atlanta, GA
Trachoma

Iván Espinoza Quinteros, MD
Assistant Professor of Pediatrics
    and Neuropediatrics
Facultad de Medicina Alberto Hurtado
Universidad Peruana Cayetano
    Heredia
Lima, Peru
Cysticercosis

Jose M. Fierro, MD, FAAP
Clinical Assistant Professor of Medicine
  and Pediatrics
University of Arizona COM
Phoenix Mountain Park Health Center
Tolleson, AZ
Malaria
Schistosomiasis

Marc Foca, MD
Assistant Professor of Clinical Pediatrics
Department of Pediatrics, Division of
  Infectious Diseases
Columbia University Medical Center
New York, NY
Tuberculosis

Samuel N. Forjuoh, MD, MPH, DrPH
Professor of Family & Community
  Medicine and Biostatistics &
  Epidemiology
Texas A&M Health Science Center,
  College of Medicine, Scott & White
Temple, TX
Burns

Jo Ann Gates, MD, FAAP
Hillsborough County Health Department
Tampa, FL
Tungiasis

Timothy E. Gibson, MD, FAAP
UMass Memorial Children's Medical
  Center
University of Massachusetts Medical
  School
Worcester, MA
Meningococcemia
Molluscum Contagiosum
Tinea
Toxoplasmosis

Marlene S. Goodfriend, MD
Clinical Assistant Professor of Pediatrics
University of Florida College of Medicine
Jacksonville, FL
Psychosocial Considerations

Ashok Gupta, MD, FIAP
Associate Professor of Pediatrics
SMS Medical College
Jaipur, India
Pyomyositis, Tropical

Julie Herlihy, MD, MPH
Pediatric Resident, Boston Combined
  Residency in Pediatrics
Children's Hospital Boston/Boston
  Medical Center
Boston, MA
Leprosy

Herminio R. Hernández Diaz
Professor of Pediatrics
Facultdad de Medicina Alberto Hurtado
Universidad Peruana Cayetano Heredia
Lima, Peru
Tuberculosis

Roger Hernández, MD
Professor of Pediatric Infectious Diseases
Universidad Peruana Cayetano Heredia
Lima, Peru
Carrion Disease
Leishmaniasis, Cutaneous

Marisa Isabel Herran, MD, FAAP
Codirector, Rainbow Center for Global
  Child Health
Assistant Professor of Pediatrics
Case Western Reserve University
Cleveland, OH
Leishmaniasis, Visceral

Donald R. Hopkins, MD, MPH
Vice President (Health)
The Carter Center
Atlanta, GA
Dracunculiasis

Lloyd R. Jensen, MD, FAAP
Assistant Clinical Professor of Pediatrics
University of Washington
Seattle, WA
Neonatal Survival

Khaliah A. Johnson, MD
Pediatric Resident, the Harriet Lane
Residency Program
Johns Hopkins Hospital Children's Center
Baltimore, MD
Pediculosis

Kirsten N. Johnson, MD, MPH
Faculty Lecturer and Attending
Physician, Departments of
Emergency & Family Medicine,
McGill University, Montreal, Canada
Faculty Fellow, Institute for Health
and Social Policy, McGill University,
Montreal Canada
Affiliated Faculty, Harvard Humanitarian
Initiative, Harvard University, Boston, MA
Dracunculiasis

Ayesha Kadir, MD
Resident Physician
University of Minnesota
Minneapolis, MN
Amebiasis
Human Rights of Children

Shiva Kalidindi, MD, MS, DTM&H
Assistant Professor of Pediatrics
Schulich School of Medicine & Dentistry
University of Western Ontario
Ontario, Canada
Cutaneous Larva Migrans

Deepak M. Kamat, MD, PhD, FAAP
Professor of Pediatrics, Wayne State
University
Vice Chair of Education
Director, Institute of Medical Education
The Carman and Ann Adams
Department of Pediatrics
Children's Hospital of Michigan
Detroit, MI
Cutaneous Larva Migrans
Mumps
Poliomyelitis
Vitamin A Deficiency

Riva Kamat-Nerikar, MD
Clinical Instructor of Pediatrics, Virginia
Commonwealth University
Inova Fairfax Hospital for Children
Falls Church, VA
Hypothyroidism, Congenital

Danielle Kauk, MD, MPH
Family Medicine Resident
Lawrence Family Medicine Residency
Lawrence, MA
Cholera

Tao Sheng Kwan-Gett, MD, MPH
Medical Epidemiologist, Public Health
Seattle & King County
Associate Clinical Professor of Pediatrics
University of Washington School
of Medicine
Seattle, WA
Rabies

Chandrakant Lahariya, MD, MBBS
Assistant Professor of Community
Medicine
G.R. Medical College and Affiliated
Hospitals
Gwalior, MP, India
Immunization in Developing Countries

Shiv Lal
Special Director General of Health
Services (Public Health)
Director, National Institute of
Communicable Diseases
Delhi, India
Chikungunya Fever

Amina Lalani, MD, FRCPC
Assistant Professor of Pediatrics
University of Toronto
Toronto, Ontario, Canada
Tetanus

Phuoc V. Le, MD, MPH
Clinical Fellow in Internal Medicine,
    Pediatrics, and Global Health Equity
Brigham and Women's Hospital
Massachusetts General Hospital
Harvard Medical School
Boston, MA
Typhoid Fever

Angela K. Lumba, MD
Department of Pediatric Emergency
    Medicine
Rady Children's Hospital, University of
    California, San Diego
San Diego, CA
Burkitt Lymphoma
Neglected Tropical Diseases
Water and Sanitation

Ciro Maguina, MD, PhD
Principal Professor of Infectious Diseases
Universidad Peruana Cayetano Heredia
Lima, Peru
Carrion Disease

**Peter MacPherson, MBChB, MPH,
    Dip, HIV(man)**
Honorary Lecturer in Public Health
University of Witwatersrand School of
    Public Health
Johannesburg, South Africa
HIV and AIDS

Anna Mandalakas, MD, MS Epi
Associate Professor of Pediatrics, Global
    & Public Health
Case Western Reserve University
Cleveland, OH
Tuberculosis

Patrick Mason, MD, PhD, FAAP
Director, International Adoption Center
Inova Fairfax Hospital for Children
Fairfax, VA
Hypothyroidism, Congenital
Rickets

Ambika Mathur, PhD
Professor of Pediatrics
Assistant Dean for Combined Degree
    Programs
Wayne State University
Detroit, MI
Vitamin A Deficiency

**Ana Luiza de Mattos Guaraldi, BSc,
    PhD**
Associate Professor of Microbiology and
    Immunology, Faculty of Medicine
University of the Rio de Janeiro
    State—UERJ
Rio de Janeiro, RJ, Brazil
Diphtheria

Peter A. Meaney, MD, MPH
Assistant Professor of Critical Care
    and Pediatrics
Specialty Director, International
    Education, Center for Simulation,
    Advanced Education and Innovation
Director, The CLEAR Initiative (Clinical
    Leadership, Education, Advocacy,
    and Research)
Children's Hospital of Philadelphia
Philadelphia, PA
Onchocerciasis

**Wayne M. Meyers, MD, PhD, DSc
    (Hon)**
Visiting Scientist
Department of Environmental and
    Infectious Disease Sciences
Armed Forces Institute of Pathology
Washington, DC
Buruli Ulcer

Veena Mittal
Joint Director and Head, Zoonosis
    Division
National Institute of Communicable
    Diseases
New Delhi, India
Chikungunya Fever

Aamir Jalal Al Mosawi, MD, PhD
Professor of Pediatrics
Head of the Department of Pediatrics
    and CME Center
University Hospital in Al Kadhimiyia
Baghdad, Iraq
Poststreptococcal Glomerulonephritis

Dena Nazer, MD
Medical Director, Child Protection
    Center
The Children's Hospital of Michigan
Assistant Professor of Pediatrics
Wayne State University
Detroit, MI
Poliomyelitis
Mumps

Brett D. Nelson, MD, MPH, DTM&H
Pediatric Global Health Fellow
Department of Pediatrics
Massachusetts General Hospital
Harvard Medical School
Boston, MA
Trypanosomiasis, African

Paula G. Newton, MD
Inova Fairfax Hospital for Children
Falls Church, VA
Rickets

**Paul N. Newton, DPhil, MRCP,
    DTM&H**
Wellcome Trust-Mahosot Hospital-
    Oxford University Tropical Medicine
    Research Collaboration
Microbiology Laboratory, Mahosot
    Hospital
Vientiane, Lao PDR
Melioidosis

Eric Nilles, MD
Assistant Professor of Emergency
    Medicine
University of Iowa
Carver College of Medicine
University of Iowa Hospital & Clinics
Iowa City, IA
Filariasis, Lymphatic

Roberto Andres Novoa, MS
Harvard Medical School
Boston, MA
Leishmaniasis, Visceral

**Winstone Nyandiko Mokaya,
    MBchB, MMED**
Senior Lecturer and Pediatrician
Department of Child Health &
    Pediatrics, School of Medicine
Moi University and Moi Teaching and
    Referral Hospital
Eldoret, Kenya
HIV and AIDS

Cliff O'Callahan, MD, PhD, FAAP
Pediatric Faculty & Director, Nurseries
Middlesex Hospital and Family Practice
    Residency
Assistant Professor of Pediatrics
University of Connecticut
Middletown, CT
Cysticercosis

Karen P. Olness, MD, FAAP
Professor of Pediatrics, Family Medicine,
    and Global Health
Case Western Reserve University
Cleveland, OH
Beriberi

B. Ryan Phelps, MD, MPH
Assistant Professor of Pediatrics, Baylor
    College of Medicine
Associate Director, Botswana-Baylor
    Children's Clinical Centre of
    Excellence
Baylor International Pediatrics AIDS
    Initiative
Gaborone, Botswana
Snakebite

Rattanphone Phetsouvanh, MD
Director of Microbiology Laboratory
Mahosot Hospital
Vientiane, Lao PDR
Melioidosis

Alan Peter Picarillo, MD, FAAP
Assistant Professor of Pediatrics
University of Massachusetts Medical
   School
Worcester, MA
Loaiasis

Françoise Portaels, PhD
Professor and Head, Mycobacteriology
   Unit
Department of Microbiology
Institute of Tropical Medicine
Antwerpen, Belgium
Buruli Ulcer

David Pugatch, MD, FAAP
Medical Director, Division of Pediatric
   Infectious Diseases
Children's Hospital Central California
Clinical Professor of Pediatrics
University of California, San Francisco-
   Fresno
Fresno, CA
HIV and AIDS

**Christopher Sanford, MD, MPH,
   DTM&H**
Clinical Assistant Professor, Department
   of Family Medicine
University of Washington
Seattle, WA
Yellow Fever

Javier Santisteban-Ponce, MD
Attending Physician, Department of
   Pediatrics
Edgardo Rebagliati National Hospital—
   EsSalud
Universidad Peruana Cayetano Heredia
Lima, Peru
Hydatid Disease
Scabies

Laura Sauvé, MD, MPH, DTM&H
Clinical Assistant Professor, Division
   of Infectious and Inflammatory
   Diseases, Department of Pediatrics
University of British Columbia
Vancouver, British Columbia, Canada
Pellagra

Charles J. Schubert, MD
Professor of Clinical Pediatrics,
   University of Cincinnati College
   of Medicine
Cincinnati Children's Hospital
   Medical Center
Cincinnati, OH
Burkitt Lymphoma

Tina M. Slusher, MD, FAAP
Associate Professor of Pediatrics
Center for Global Pediatrics
University of Minnesota
Minneapolis, MN
Measles

Christopher C. Stewart, MD, MA
Assistant Professor of Pediatrics
University of California, San Francisco
San Francisco, CA
Ascariasis

M. Leila Srour, MD, MPH, DTM&H
Health Frontiers
Vientiane, Lao PDR
Noma

Jürg Utzinger, PhD
Tenure-Track Associate Professor of
   Epidemiology
Department of Public Health and
   Epidemiology
Swiss Tropical Institute
Basel, Switzerland
Schistosomiasis

Rohitkumar Vasa, MD, FAAP
Director of Neonatology, Mercy Hospital and Medical Center
Clinical Associate, University of Chicago
Chicago, IL
Traditional Health Practices

Eduardo Verne, MD
Professor of Pediatric Infectious Diseases
Universidad Peruana Cayetano Heredia
Lima, Peru
Cysticercosis
Varicella-Zoster and Herpes Zoster Infections

Ung Vibol, MD
Head of TB/HIV Department, National Pediatric Hospital
Lecturer for University of Health Science
Phnom Penh
Cambodia
HIV and AIDS

Rais Vohra, MD
Assistant Professor of Emergency Medicine
Director of Toxicology
Olive View-UCLA Medical Center
David Geffen School of Medicine
Los Angeles, CA
Snakebite

Annie R. Wang
Warren Alpert Medical School of Brown University
Providence, RI
HIV and AIDS

Table of Contents

Introduction

This atlas, which during development evolved to become a true global collaborative effort, was born from the idea that educational messages shared through the right visual information can facilitate a powerful process of rapid and sustained learning. We hope that health care workers' enhanced understanding of child illness will catalyze a process of improved care for children and their families living in tropical and resource-limited settings worldwide.

Many conditions described in this text are inexorably linked to population health concerns, and deliberate attempts were made to address these important relationships wherever possible. The first section of this book attends specifically to pressing issues in international public health. The second section then describes individual pathologic states in greater detail. Given the considerable burden of global child illness attributable to nutritional disease, it seemed appropriate to further equip readers with essential tools used to diagnose malnutrition. To that end, a mid-upper arm circumference (MUAC) band and weight-for-height tables are included. Also found in the appendices is a table of common therapeutic regimens for diseases discussed in the book.

We are grateful to friends and colleagues who worked with us at the American Academy of Pediatrics (AAP) Section on International Child Health to produce this atlas. Particular appreciation goes to the contributing editors and authors; Javier Santisteban-Ponce and his team at the Gorgas Institute of Tropical Medicine in Lima, Peru; Mark Taylor and the Liverpool School of Tropical Medicine; Juerg Utzinger and the Swiss Tropical Institute; Jeremy Green and the International Trachoma Institute; Bryan Watt Humanitarian Photography; Paige Rohe; The Carter Center; the Mectizan Donation Program; Jorge Atouguia and the Instituto de Higiene e Medicina Tropical in Lisbon, Portugal; Holger Brockmeyer; Larry Schwab; Manson Publishing Ltd, London; Office of Medical History and Office of the Surgeon General, US Army; AMPATH, Kenya; Stephen Figge; Doctors Without Borders/ Médecins Sans Frontières (MSF); the World Health Organization; Martha Cook; Mark Grimes; Maureen DeRosa; and the AAP Department of Marketing and Publications. In addition, we are thankful for the existence of several extremely high-quality resources including the AAP *Red Book*; MSF Clinical Guidelines; Gill and Beeching's *Lecture Notes on Tropical Medicine*; Guerrant, Walker, and Weller's *Essentials of Tropical Infectious Diseases*; Michele Barry's *New England Journal of Medicine* guinea worm review; and the Centers for Disease Control and Prevention Public Health Image Library.

Please note that a portion of revenues from the sale of the book will fund meaningful programs in global health sponsored by the AAP Section on International Child Health.

Your partnership is vital to enriching future editions of this atlas. We welcome your comments and contributions at jmspector@aap.net.

J. Spector
T. Gibson
Cambridge 2009

Human Rights of Children

BACKGROUND

Proper assessment of tropical diseases affecting children is not complete without addressing the issue of human rights and its relevance to health and well-being. A welcome discourse exists regarding the social aspects of disease and the clinical implications of social, political, and economic ailments. The effects of poverty on child development, morbidity, and mortality have been well documented. Still, 10 million children younger than 5 years die from treatable conditions each year. More than a quarter of these deaths occur during the neonatal period and another half are related to undernutrition. The lamentable state of many of the world's children results largely from economic and social conditions that engender ill health. These conditions include, but are not limited to, poor nutrition, lack of potable water and sanitation, education deficiencies, physical labor, proximity to violent conflict, insufficient preventive care, and limited means by which to bring these injustices into the view of the more fortunate. Health and human rights are intimately related, and the health of children cannot be viewed outside the context of human rights.

UNIVERSAL DECLARATION ON HUMAN RIGHTS

Article 25 of the United Nations' Universal Declaration on Human Rights, first signed in 1948, states that all humans have "the right to a standard of living adequate for the health and well-being of himself and of his family, including food, clothing, housing and medical care and necessary social services, and the right to security in the event of unemployment, sickness, disability, widowhood, old age or other lack of livelihood in circumstances beyond his control." Concern for women and children is specifically addressed: "Motherhood and childhood are entitled to special care and assistance. All children, whether born in or out of wedlock, shall enjoy the same social protection."

The right to a name, to citizenship, and to "the conditions that allow for a standard of living adequate for health and well-being" may at first glance seem obvious, but the evidence shows that much of the world lives without some, most, or all of these rights. Structural violence refers to the social, political, and economic conditions that prevent a person from living up to his or her full potential, and in extreme cases, from meeting basic needs. It is the structure of the society that is violent, as factors such as racism, gender inequality, and wealth and health disparities ensure that disadvantaged people are disproportionately more likely to come to harm. The implication is that, under a different social arrangement, the injuries sustained would be prevented. Ultimately, structural violence dictates the choices an individual is given throughout life as well as the kinds of choices that person will make. Thus the poor are more likely to suffer from intestinal helminths, cholera, or tuberculosis; live in slums; receive little or no schooling; start work at a young age; be sold into slavery; contract HIV; and turn to violence or crime as a means of subsistence.

COLLECTIVE RESPONSIBILITY

As physicians and health care professionals, we see firsthand the effects of structural violence on the lives of our patients. Those who practice in developed countries know that poor children are less likely to follow through with well-child checks or to receive immunizations; they are more likely to drop out of school, be overweight, join a gang, or be incarcerated. Health care workers in developing countries know that poor children are more likely to suffer from chronic and acute malnutrition, receive little schooling, be orphaned, be displaced, start work at an early age, and die prematurely. For children, the human right to health and well-being necessitates the health and well-being of those who care for them. Thus to realize the rights of children, one must also realize the rights of their caregivers and to work for the well-being of the entire society. Because poor children and their caregivers have neither the voice nor power to make known the injustices they endure, it is the responsibility of those who work with them, those who are witness to the injustices they endure, to learn about these injustices and to work to eradicate them.

There is a growing multidisciplinary body of literature on the reciprocity between clinical medicine, social medicine, public health, and human rights. While this development is positive and inherently proactive, the flurry of data and rhetoric has remained confined to a small group of highly interested individuals, and has yet to penetrate the mainstream medical and social academic professions. Working for human rights has until recently been looked on as outside the scope of pediatric practice. But today, the growing knowledge of environmental factors on health and the role of structural violence in the lives of the poor have made something as apparently simple as the right to health a requisite to good pediatric care.

Immunization in Developing Countries

BACKGROUND

The first vaccine, targeting smallpox, was discovered in the late 1700s—it was not until almost 2 centuries later that immunization services began to reach children in low-income countries. The World Health Organization (WHO) and UNICEF proposed the Expanded Programme on Immunization in 1974 with the goal of universal coverage by 1990. Unfortunately, this challenge has not yet been met. Immunization, perhaps the most effective public health intervention in history, is underutilized in developing regions. While an estimated 2.5 million deaths are averted each year by vaccination, 2 million children still die from diseases entirely preventable by vaccines recommended by the WHO, and an additional 2 million lives could be saved if vaccines for pathogens such as rotavirus, meningococcus, and pneumococcus were widely distributed.

WHAT, WHERE, AND WHY

There is reason for optimism. Overall, vaccine coverage has increased in recent years. More than 150 countries reported diphtheria, pertussis, and tetanus immunization coverage rates of 80% or greater in 2006. Approximately 90% of countries provide measles immunization. Smallpox has been eradicated and polio and tetanus have been virtually eliminated in many parts of the world.

The problem is that a considerable percentage of populations continue to suffer from limited access to immunizations, and the gap in coverage between well and poorly performing nations may be widening. Twenty-six million children are not protected against diphtheria, pertussis, and tetanus. Polio continues to be endemic in 4 countries. Newer vaccines have extremely low coverage rates in certain regions. Themes for disparities in immunization coverage across the globe are similar to those that result in other health and development inequalities. Poor access to health facilities and immunization campaigns, deficient resources, lack of political will, civil conflict and war, and natural disasters all contribute. Logistical concerns relating to vaccine distribution are an additional crucial factor since refrigeration is required throughout vaccine transport, which sometimes occurs in blisteringly hot environments. Not surprisingly, most vaccine-preventable illness is found in less developed countries, particularly those in sub-Saharan African, Asia, the Middle East, and Central and South America.

RECENT DEVELOPMENTS

Growing appreciation for timely distribution of immunizations has helped to pave the way for dissemination of newer vaccines, including those against hepatitis B (HBV) and *Haemophilus influenzae* type b (Hib). Their introduction has been supported by powerful international organizations such as the Global Alliance for Vaccines and Immunization, which helps supply vaccines to resource-limited settings. In the past, distribution of new vaccines to developing countries was delayed on average by 15 years relative to industrialized nations. Now, many low-income countries are breaking this pattern and becoming early adopters. Nearly 150 countries have introduced HBV and Hib into their national immunization programs. Other vaccines, including those against typhoid, pneumococcal disease, and rotavirus infection, may soon follow this precedent.

THE WAY FORWARD

The vital importance of immunizations in reducing the burden of vaccine-preventable disease is well recognized. Immunization coverage with traditional EPI vaccines is increasing in many parts of the world, and developing countries are also adopting newer vaccines. Still, much work has yet to be done to ensure widespread coverage and to prevent avoidable disease in all of the world's children. International groups must continue to work closely with local partners and governments to guarantee constructive political advocacy, provide technical and funding support, and further build capacity of national immunization programs.

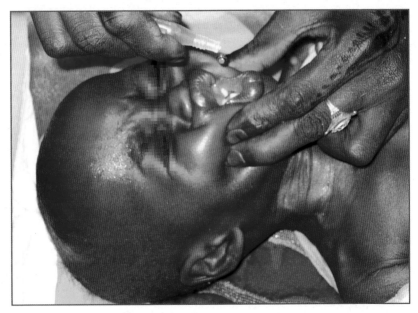

IMAGE 1
Drops of oral polio vaccine, costing less than a few pennies, prevent lifelong morbidity or death.

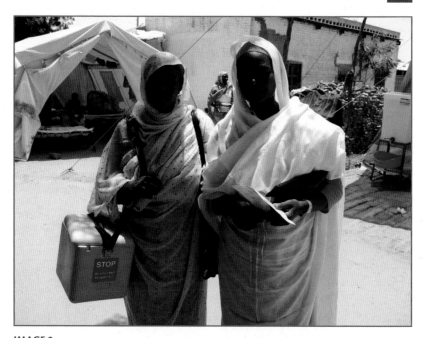

IMAGE 2

Maintaining an effective cold chain from vaccine production to the site of ultimate administration constitutes one of the greatest logistical challenges to universal immunization. The Ministry of Health immunization outreach workers shown here are carrying a cold box filled with vaccine vials.

Neglected Tropical Diseases

So-called neglected tropical diseases are endemic to certain impoverished areas of the tropical world and are collectively responsible for enormous morbidity, often because of poor capacity for prevention and inadequate access to treatment. These conditions are largely absent from wealthy societies and are not typically associated with outbreaks that might capture the attention of the global community. Those most affected often live in remote areas of low-income countries and lack the ability to advocate on their own behalf for health care or public health improvements. Despite the great disability and death they cause, neglected tropical diseases are effectively hidden from much of the world—they are not addressed by governments of endemic countries because of financial or political constraints, and international assistance is insufficient.

The World Health Organization (WHO) estimates that as of 2008, approximately 1 billion people have one or more of these diseases. Many illnesses fall under the umbrella of neglected tropical diseases. Currently, the WHO lists the following 14: Buruli ulcer, Chagas disease, cholera/epidemic diarrhea diseases, dengue/dengue hemorrhagic fever, dracunculiasis (guinea worm), endemic treponematoses (yaws, pinta, endemic syphilis), human African trypanosomiasis (sleeping sickness), leishmaniasis, leprosy, lymphatic filariasis, onchocerciasis, schistosomiasis, soil-transmitted helminthiasis, and trachoma.

Neonatal Survival

BACKGROUND

Nearly 4 million babies die each year in the neonatal period (the first 4 weeks of life), primarily from preventable causes in resource-constrained settings. Stillbirths likely account for several million additional deaths. Given that global mortality for children younger than 5 years is estimated at nearly 10 million, the burden of disease among children that is attributable to neonatal illness is grossly disproportionate. Moreover, while overall child survival has improved in the past few decades, neonatal mortality rates in many countries have remained stable or even increased. The worldwide neonatal mortality rate average is 30 deaths per 1,000 live births. It is now well recognized that United Nations' Millennium Development Goal 4 (calling for reduction by two-thirds in child mortality from 1990 to 2015) will not be achieved without successfully targeting newborn disease.

WHERE, WHEN, AND WHY

Regional discrepancies in neonatal mortality are considerable. Ninety-nine percent of neonatal deaths occur in less developed parts of the world where home births are common. While neonatal mortality rates in industrialized countries are on the order of 5 per 1,000 live births, many regions of Africa, Asia, and the Middle East have rates above 45 per 1,000 live births. A newborn in Africa is 8 times more likely to die than her counterpart born in the United Kingdom.

Of babies dying in the first month of life, approximately two-thirds die in the first week, and two-thirds of those die in the first 24 hours. The first minutes following delivery, during which time many babies need assistance transitioning to life outside the uterus, can be particularly precarious. The 3 major causes of neonatal mortality are infections, birth asphyxia, and complications related to prematurity. Low-birth-weight babies constitute 15% of births and contribute to 60% to 80% of mortality. Neonatal tetanus, a completely preventable condition, continues to account for more than a quarter-million deaths annually.

TREATMENT AND PREVENTION

Integrating beneficial newborn care practices into existing community health systems is vital for both prevention and management of neonatal disease. Major elements of essential newborn care put forth by the World Health Organization include ensuring clean delivery and cord care, provision of effective neonatal resuscitation practices, thermal protection, early and exclusive breastfeeding, antibiotic eye prophylaxis, immunization, special attention to preterm and low-birth-weight infants, and timely recognition of newborn illness followed by referral when necessary.

Home- and community-based neonatal care programs are of critical importance to caring for families that lack access to health facilities.

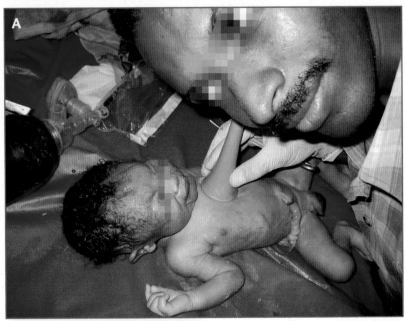

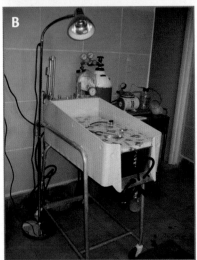

IMAGE 1A, 1B

Ten percent of newborns require assistance at the time of birth. Neonatal resuscitation can be a life-saving practice for babies who fail to initiate spontaneous breathing. This infant was delivered urgently to a mother suffering from eclampsia, and remained apneic and cyanotic until a few manual breaths with a bag and mask were delivered (Image 1A). Afterward, the baby did well. Accurate case reporting is difficult in many settings, and this infant might have inappropriately been labeled a stillbirth had he not survived. An example of a resuscitation area in a rural birthing center shows heating and suction devices, and an Ambu-Bag (Image 1B).

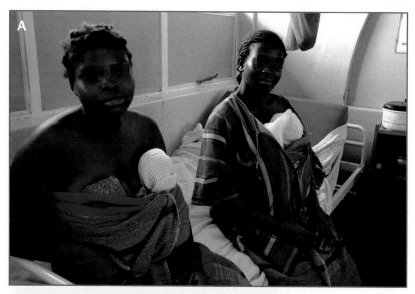

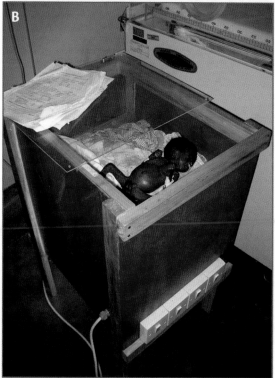

IMAGE 2A, 2B
Hypothermia is a preventable contributor to neonatal morbidity and mortality, especially in premature and low-birth-weight infants. Childbirth should take place in warm rooms that are free from cooling drafts, newborns should be quickly dried, and bathing should be delayed to prevent unnecessary heat loss. Skin-to-skin contact with the mother (sometimes called *kangaroo mother care*) is frequently encouraged (Image 2A). In health facilities, incubators may be useful management adjuncts. The model depicted was made locally in Malawi from wood and lightbulbs (Image 2B).

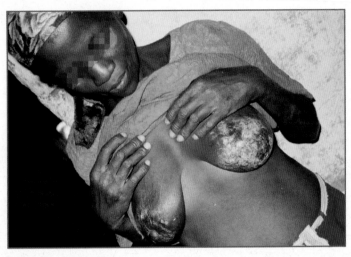

IMAGE 3

The effect of exclusive breastfeeding on newborn and infant health is striking. Mortality rates of non-breastfed neonates are up to 7-fold greater than of those who are breastfed. Populations in industrialized countries may take for granted the wide availability of safe, alternative formulas. In many poorer communities, breastfeeding difficulties (as occurs, for example, with maternal mastitis) correlate with newborn illness and death.

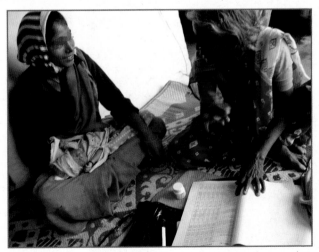

IMAGE 4

Abhay and Rani Bang, with their team in Gadchiroli, India, have demonstrated that a home-based neonatal care package can lead to dramatic improvements in newborn survival. Here, a community health worker interviews a mother about her 10-day-old infant. She will measure the baby's vital signs and perform a physical examination. In the event that infection is suspected, parenteral antibiotics can be administered. *Courtesy: Society for Education, Action and Research in Community Health (SEARCH).*

Psychosocial Considerations

BACKGROUND

Understanding the psychosocial milieu of children is critical to providing care that promotes the highest level of growth, development, and overall well-being. It follows then that pediatric practice in less developed settings must be delivered in the context of a thorough awareness of the region's historical background, the family's life, and child development. Psychosocial handicaps can result from countless risks, including those relating to physiological (eg, nutrient deficiency), familial (eg, death of parent), cultural (eg, harmful traditional practices), and societal (eg, civil conflict) concerns. Up to 200 million children younger than 5 years who live in resource-limited parts of the world fail to reach their full cognitive potential, and many millions more may be psychologically or emotionally stunted.

Physical and psychosocial environments affect the behavior and development of infants and children. The home setting is an essential consideration. When evaluating children, it might be useful to know, for instance, if the parents work, whether children are schooled or working, if children are separated from their mothers during the day, or whether the family is economically stable. An assessment of the types of stimulation that are available and administered is vital for children of all ages.

EFFECT OF MALNUTRITION

Malnutrition is a leading cause of global morbidity and constitutes a major risk factor for poor child development. Breakdown of parent-child relationships may be noted in affected families, and comprehensive evaluation of malnourished children must incorporate a full account of caregiver capacity and function. Malnourished children can be challenging to care for, and even loving mothers and fathers can become discouraged, feel helpless, and withdraw from their children. Moreover, primary caretakers may often not be the biological parents, who might be ill, have left the family, or have passed away. World Health Organization guidelines specifically address the importance of psychosocial stimulation when managing children with malnutrition.

ANTICIPATING AND INTERVENING

Country histories, encompassing both recent and distant past, profoundly affect a population's psyche. Natural disasters such as earthquakes or tsunamis may have resulted in loss of life, homes, or priceless possessions. Families displaced by conflict are uniformly stressed and traumatized. In response, children and their families can suffer anxiety and post-traumatic stress disorders. Sleeping difficulties, nightmares, hyperarousal, excessive fear, clinging, crying, dysphoria, and flashbacks are not uncommon. Parents may benefit from guidance in recognizing and accepting the root of these symptoms, and learning techniques for reassuring, calming, and stabilizing their children and themselves.

Thoughtful speech, motor, cognitive, and behavioral evaluations are central to implementing changes that positively influence developmental, learning, and social progress. The first 3 years of life are a particularly crucial period for brain development. Early intervention is key. A paucity of formal preventive and therapeutic programs exist in the developing world, and it is therefore incumbent on health care workers to identify developmental delays and guide therapy whenever possible.

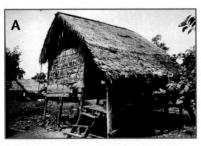
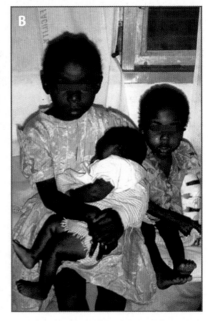

IMAGE 1A, 1B
Psychosocial development is influenced by the physical environment. Many people living in a small house can lead to persistent noise and an atmosphere of disorganization (Image 1A). Infants, especially those born premature or with low birth weights, may consequently exhibit irritability or other behavioral problems. Not uncommonly, mothers in tropical regions work during the day and leave their children in the care of other children (Image 1B). Pica, a condition associated with maternal deprivation and low socioeconomic status, may be seen in these populations. *Courtesy: Marlene Goodfriend.*

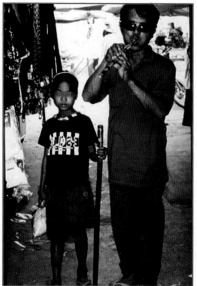

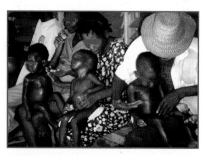

IMAGE 3

Culturally appropriate and easy-to-perform practices are the most successful and sustainable interventions. Parents massaging and singing to malnourished Haitian children promote positive interactions and create a sense of well-being in both the parents and the children. *Courtesy: Marlene Goodfriend.*

IMAGE 2

A country's past affects the care of children in the present. The young girl shown is caring for her father who was blinded by a land mine explosion. Pediatric practice in Cambodia, for example, necessitates an understanding of the dramatic impact of the Khmer Rouge. Many parents who survived the bloody regime witnessed the deaths of family members and were noted to be overly anxious when their children developed minor medical illnesses. Having experienced much death, families were fearful for the lives of their children. Health care workers also discovered that parents did not want their children to wear eyeglasses, which was perceived as a symbol of intelligence, because the region's intelligentsia had been viciously persecuted. *Courtesy: Marlene Goodfriend.*

Traditional Health Practices

BACKGROUND

Traditional medicine generally refers to healing practices based on cultural or religious beliefs, often endorsed by elders or other community authorities who were themselves trained by prior generations. The terms *unconventional, complementary,* and *alternative* are also variably used and meant to distinguish traditional healing from *conventional, evidence-based, Western,* or *modern* modes of medicine in which therapies have presumably been formally evaluated (ie, through clinical trials).

While traditional medicine in some form is practiced considerably in industrialized countries (eg, among as much as 40%–60% of populations in the United Kingdom and United States), its use in less well-developed regions appears to be even greater. Moreover, while these practices are often truly complementary in resource-rich communities, they many times represent primary care in austere settings.

A number of factors influence the widespread adoption of traditional health practice in resource-constrained parts of the world, including restricted accessibility to conventional practitioners, medicines, and supplies; financial concerns; educational limitations; and support of local remedies by respected community members.

INTEGRATIVE MEDICINE

Most governments, at some level, show consideration for the paradigms intrinsic to traditional health systems, but the extent to which these practices are recognized in national health policies is varied. Integrative medicine combines elements of traditional and conventional care. This approach is taken, for instance, in parts of India, China, and Thailand, where many traditional healing techniques have been officially sanctioned, local practitioners receive certified training, and traditional medical practice is an accepted and legal activity. Other controlling bodies are less sympathetic to medical practice perceived as unconventional and either tolerate parallel care systems or forbid them.

FIELD PRACTICE

Scarification, cupping, tattooing, and concoction application or ingestion are examples of healing techniques associated with traditional medicine, but the list of existing practices is long, diverse, and context dependent. Health care professionals should become knowledgeable about the cultural and spiritual commonalities that are prevalent within the communities they serve, and understand which practices are officially permitted and which might be unlawful. Many find it helpful to develop their own assessment of traditional remedies and categorize them as useful, innocuous, harmful, or of uncertain utility. An important consideration is the ethical quandary that may arise when deferral to local customs precludes conventional treatment. This is of particular concern when traditional medical practice risks delay in conventional care-seeking for a child with a major illness. Cultivating meaningful partnerships with colleagues in the field can go far toward developing a rational method for respecting traditional healing while ensuring optimal care for children and families.

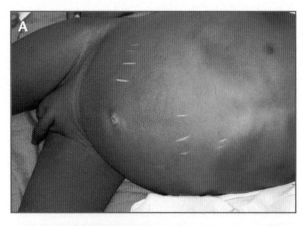

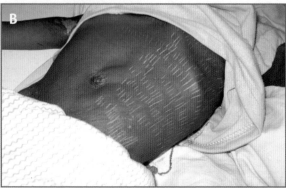

IMAGE 1A, 1B

Scarification exemplifies a traditional healing technique frequently not condoned by conventional practitioners who consider the practice unproven, painful, and potentially harmful. The Sudanese child seen in Image 1B was extremely ill on arrival at the district hospital and, given the considerable number of lesions, his physicians wondered whether reliance on traditional medicine had delayed his presentation.

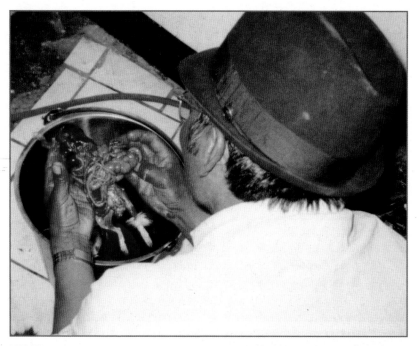

IMAGE 2

In the Ecuadorian Highlands, traditional healers known as *Yachacs* perform *una limpia de cuy* (literally, guinea pig cleansing). It is said that chanting and shaking the animal around the patient transmits disease from child to *cuy*. The rodent is then sacrificed, dissected, and examined to determine the diagnosis. *Courtesy: Stephanie Doniger.*

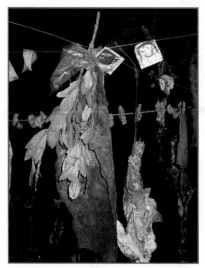

IMAGE 3

In collaboration with local health care programs, a traditional healer in South Africa advertises and dispenses condoms alongside traditional medicine to promote HIV prevention in the community. *Courtesy: Keri Cohn.*

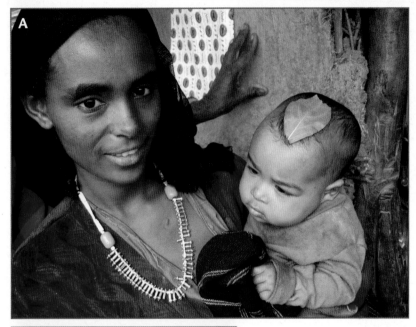

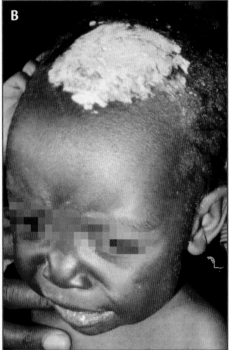

IMAGE 4A, 4B
Conventional wisdom often ascribes sunken fontanels in infants to conditions such as dehydration. Local understandings of disease may lead to alternative treatment regimens, such as covering the area with a leaf or even food products.

Water and Sanitation

BACKGROUND

History is replete with episodes of devastating disease promoted by waste materials. The *Yersinia pestis* plague of the 14th century and the tragedy of cholera, famously depicted by Gabriel Garcia Marquez, are dramatic examples of the reality that many millions of children endure—health consequences of inadequate hygiene. Contaminated water and poor sanitation represent the catalyst and mechanism of infection by which a massive burden of tropical illness is produced.

Several key enablers facilitate transmission of tropical disease. Tropical climates typically range from 80°F to 90°F with frequent rainfall, which aids rapid multiplication and spread of organisms in the absence of proper sanitation. Lush environments are optimal for the survival of pathogens, animals and their zoonoses, and insect vectors of disease. Poverty contributes to poor hygiene because of crowded living conditions and limited preventive resources. Improper food storage and disposal with subsequent invasion of animals and insects compound the spread of infection via fecal-oral routes. This problem is magnified in the tropics where food spoils quickly and bacteria thrive. Natural water supplies can easily be contaminated by human or animal waste, sewage, and wastewater run-off. Moreover, the warm waters of tropical climates, which may be used as drinking water, are ideal for direct inhabitation and propagation of parasites. The cycle of daily life in many communities inadvertently, but directly, propagates the spread of disease. Issues related to water and sanitation are thought to be responsible for nearly 90% of global diarrheal illness. Most deaths caused by diarrhea occur in children younger than 5 years (see Box 1).

EPIDEMIOLOGY

According to the World Health Organization (WHO), greater than 2 billion people lack access to adequate sanitation facilities and 1 billion people do not have clean water supplies. More than half live in Asia, particularly China and India. Populations in sub-Saharan Africa are also considerably affected.

SOLUTIONS

Education is critical in effecting positive changes in hygiene and other behaviors associated with disease spread. Encouraging hand-washing after possible contact with feces is a simple but crucial practice that aids disease prevention. Establishing functional latrines is important, especially in resource-constrained communities, where the lack of

Box 1. Examples of Disease Perpetuated by Contaminated Water

Bacteria	Viruses	Helminths and Protozoa
Escherichia coli	Norovirus	Dracunculi
Salmonella sp.	Rotavirus	Schistosoma
Shigella sp.	Hepatitis A	*Cryptosporidium parvum*
Yersinia enterocolitica	Adenovirus	*Giardia lamblia*
Campylobacter sp.	Astrovirus	Leishmania
Vibrio sp.	Calicivirus	Trypanosoma sp.
Leptospira sp.	Poliovirus	*Entamoeba histolytica*
Brucella sp.	Polyomavirus	*Taenia solium*
Legionella	Coronavirus	Cyclospora
	Dengue fever	Microsporidia
	Hemorrhagic fevers	Plasmodium sp. (malaria)
	Yellow fever	Ascaris sp.
	Dengue fever	

designated areas for defecation potentiate contamination of water and soil. Waste sites should be located away from living areas and watershed paths. Reducing the collection of stagnant waters can help to decrease the spread of vector-borne disease. Sources of drinking water must be completely separate from bathing or sewage facilities and, if possible, chlorinated. Water should be boiled before consumption if clean water is unobtainable. Seemingly small changes in daily life can significantly impact disease transmission.

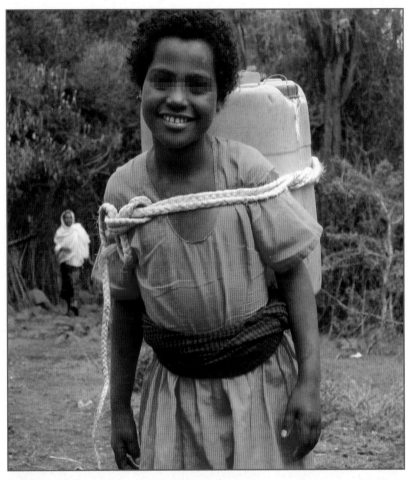

IMAGE 1

A young Ethiopian girl embarks on her daily chore: transport of 20 kg of water from stream to home. The natural water source itself may contain pathogenic organisms, even without human contamination.

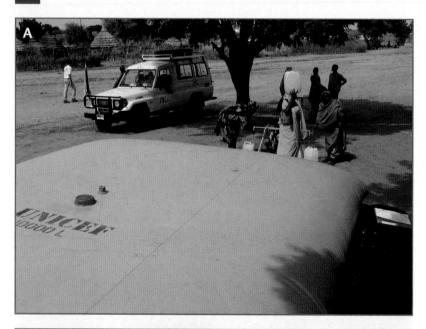

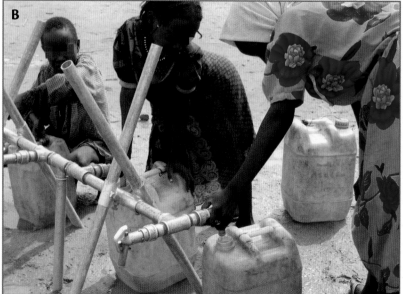

IMAGE 2A, 2B

Ensuring availability of sufficient quantities of potable water to populations affected by complex humanitarian crises can be logistically challenging. In this context, water is sometimes chemically treated in large bladders and piped to easily accessed spigots.

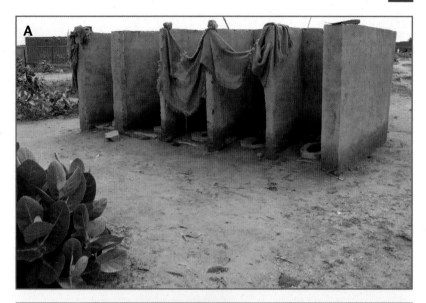

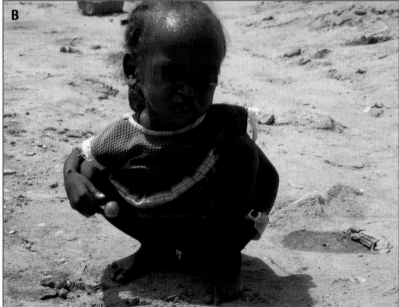

IMAGE 3A, 3B

Pit latrines are essential for preventing the spread of disease caused by human waste, particularly in crowded settings such as refugee or IDP (internally displaced person) camps. Still, those not used to using such structures may be hesitant to do so. This is especially true for young children, who might be scared to enter latrines that are typically dark, enclosed, and have a big hole.

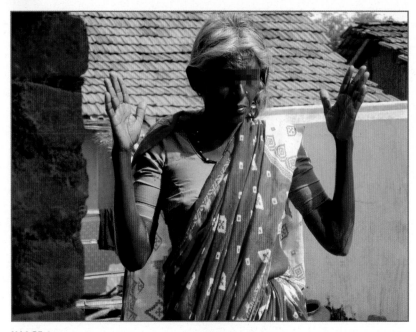

IMAGE 4

A village health worker in India washes her hands before examining a newborn, but the only clean place to dry them is in the hot sun. *Courtesy: Abhay Bang, Society for Education, Action, and Research in Community Health (SEARCH).*

Amebiasis

BACKGROUND

Entamoeba histolytica infects hundreds of millions of people each year. Of these, an estimated 50 million people develop invasive disease and 100,000 die, making *E histolytica* the third-leading cause of death from parasitic disease in the developing world. Disease is prevalent worldwide, but is most common in tropical areas, where up to 50% of inhabitants in some regions are infected with *E histolytica* or the nonpathogenic and morphologically indistinguishable strain *Entamoeba dispar*. The heaviest burden of disease is carried among people of low socioeconomic status. Clinical presentation generally varies by location. For example, dysentery is predominant in Egypt, and liver abscess is seen more frequently in South Africa and Vietnam. Children with fulminant invasive disease have the highest mortality rates, particularly when disease is compounded by undernutrition or coinfection with other diarrhea-causing pathogens.

PATHOPHYSIOLOGY

E histolytica is acquired after ingestion of infected cysts from fecally contaminated food or water. Excystation occurs in the lumen of the small bowel, and trophozoites migrate to the colonic wall where they attach to mucins and replicate. The life cycle is completed when cysts are produced and excreted. An estimated 90% of infected individuals are asymptomatic. Resistance to severe infection depends primarily on the humoral immune system and nonimmune host defenses such as intact colonic mucosa.

Disease occurs when trophozoites escape the intestinal lumen, penetrate the mucin layer, and attach to colonic wall glycoproteins to cause colitis. Further penetration through the disrupted colonic epithelial layer results in the proteolysis and cytolysis that leads to invasive disease. Gross findings range from nonspecific colonic mucosal thickening to classically described flask-shaped ulcers. Chronic symptoms and ulceration can mimic inflammatory bowel disease.

Liver abscess occurs when amebas ascend the portal venous system, causing necrosis with formation of microabscesses, which then coalesce to form larger abscesses. Ischemic hepatic necrosis results

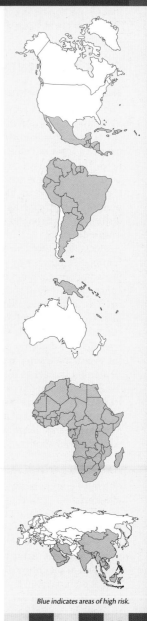

Blue indicates areas of high risk.

from obstruction of the portal vessels, periportal inflammation, and fibrosis. Other extraintestinal manifestations include peritonitis, empyema, lung abscess, brain abscess, and genitourinary disease.

CLINICAL PRESENTATION

Intestinal Amebiasis

The most common presentation of E histolytica infection is frequent, loose stools and abdominal pain occurring over 1 to 3 weeks in the absence of fever. The liver may be enlarged and tender. While stools are not usually grossly bloody, occult blood is often present. Dehydration and electrolyte disturbances are possible in those with severe diarrhea.

Rectal bleeding, chronic colitis, and fulminant colitis are other possible presentations. Children with fulminant colitis are acutely ill with fever, abdominal pain, and profuse bloody mucoid diarrhea. Such patients are at higher risk for intestinal perforation, sepsis, liver abscess, and colonic necrosis. In the event of intestinal perforation and peritonitis, corrective surgical options are limited due to difficulty suturing friable and necrotic intestinal mucosa. Other complications of acute colitis include perianal ulceration, toxic megacolon, and ameboma.

Extraintestinal Amebiasis

The most common extraintestinal manifestation of amebiasis is hepatic abscess formation. Amebic liver abscess presents acutely or subacutely, or can be a self-limiting condition with few or no symptoms. Acute onset presents with dull or pleuritic right upper quadrant abdominal pain and transient fever. Subacute disease often manifests with weight loss. Half of patients have fever and one-third have diarrhea. Dullness,

rales at the right lung base, and nonproductive cough suggest an associated pleural effusion or atelectasis. The liver is very tender, but only enlarged in half of patients. Jaundice and peritoneal signs are uncommon and indicate the presence of serious, complicated disease.

DIAGNOSTIC METHODS

The mainstay of diagnosis in many settings continues to be stool microscopy. Specimens should be fixed, stained, and examined for cysts or trophozoites within 30 minutes of collection. Note that this technique does not differentiate between infection with E histolytica and E dispar. Serum antiamebic antibodies usually appear in patients with symptoms of at least 7 days' duration. In more sophisticated centers, diagnosis can be made by serum and stool antigen testing; serology; polymerase chain reaction; and, in select cases, by colonoscopy with microscopy of biopsy samples.

Amebic liver abscess is diagnosed based on clinical presentation, epidemiological risk factors, serologic testing, and imaging. Abdominal ultrasound usually suffices. Computed tomography may be helpful in some patients. Fine-needle aspiration has low yield.

TREATMENT AND PREVENTION

Amebic colitis is treated with metronidazole or tinidazole in conjunction with an intraluminal agent such as iodoquinol or paromomycin.

Because amebic infection is most often spread through contaminated food and water, the best approach to prevent infection is to eradicate fecal contamination of food and water, improve waste disposal, reduce overcrowding, create water purification systems in endemic areas, and ensure access to clean water sources.

Education programs in endemic areas should stress the importance of hand hygiene, boiling water before consumption, and cleaning fresh foods. Vaccine production is in development and, together with efforts to improve health care, standards of living, and access to clean water, could make a substantial impact on morbidity and mortality in the developing world.

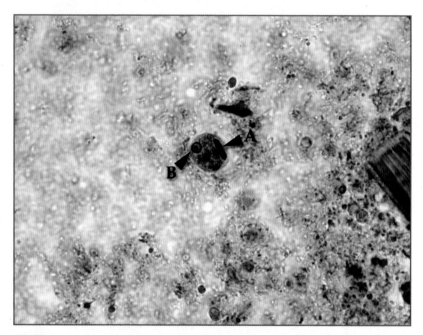

IMAGE 1

Infective cyst forms of the single-celled parasite *Entamoeba histolytica* are extremely resilient and can survive independently for many weeks. Note the presence of an elongated, blunt-ended chromatoid body within the cyst (arrow A) and a well-defined nucleus (arrow B). *Courtesy: Centers for Disease Control and Prevention/Melanie Moser.*

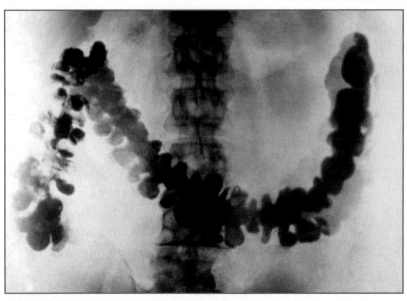

IMAGE 2

Colonic amebiasis can be suggested by contrast radiography. *Courtesy: Centers for Disease Control and Prevention/Mae Melvin and E. West.*

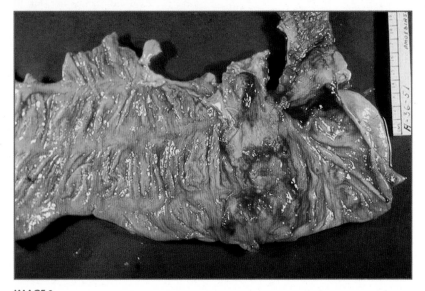

IMAGE 3

Gross pathology of intestinal amebiasis reveals extensive ulceration. *Courtesy: Centers for Disease Control and Prevention/Mae Melvin and E. West.*

Ancylostomiasis

COMMON NAME

Hookworm

BACKGROUND

Ancylostomiasis is caused by the roundworms *Necator americanus* and *Ancylostoma duodenale*. More than 700 million people worldwide are affected. While most infections are asymptomatic, hookworm remains a significant cause of anemia and malnutrition among children in the developing world. *N americanus* is the commonest hookworm in the Americas and Australia, whereas *A duodenale* is endemic in the Middle East, Southern Europe, and North Africa. Both species are found in sub-Saharan Africa and Asia. Adolescent girls and women of childbearing age are at particularly high risk for morbidity from ancylostomiasis. Their high rates of anemia are thought to result from a complex interaction of hookworm infection with nutritional and hormonal effects.

PATHOPHYSIOLOGY

Humans acquire hookworm following cutaneous penetration by infective larvae. Parasites travel hematogenously to the heart and lungs, migrate through alveoli, and ascend the bronchial tree by ciliary action. Worms are swallowed and attach themselves to the mucosa of the small intestine, where they mature. The total journey averages 1 week. Bloodsucking of the intestinal lining causes characteristic anemia. The adult worm life span is generally 1 to 2 years, during which time many thousands of eggs are passed each day in stool. Rhabditiform larvae are released from eggs and mature in soil, where they can survive for weeks. Larvae life span is longest in dry, sandy soil at temperatures in the range of 20°C to 30°C.

CLINICAL PRESENTATION

Pruritis (or ground itch) sometimes occurs when filariform larvae penetrate skin. Larval migration through the respiratory tract may trigger cough, sore throat, and fever. However, true Löffler syndrome (paroxysmal cough, dyspnea, and eosinophilia during pulmonary migration) is less common than with ascariasis. Blood

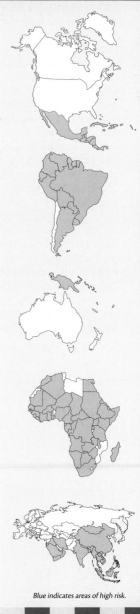

Blue indicates areas of high risk.

31

loss is proportionate to worm burden and can lead to significant iron deficiency anemia. Pallor often develops with moderate disease. Progressive anemia may result in cardiovascular complications with shortness of breath and early fatigue. Nonspecific gastrointestinal symptoms are common. Nutritional and metabolic effects occur frequently, especially in the context of coinfection with other parasites. Ingestion of a large number of *A duodenale* eggs risks development of Wakana disease, characterized by dramatic nausea, vomiting, and shortness of breath. Chronic infection is associated with growth retardation, developmental delay, and school absenteeism.

DIAGNOSIS

Stool examination yields typical hookworm ova, usually visible 1 to 3 months following initial infection. Techniques such as Wisconsin flotation and simple gravity sedimentation aid in maximizing sensitivity. Worm burden can be estimated by counting the number of eggs per gram of stool, multiplying by the daily stool weight, and dividing the result by 25,000. Infections with fewer than 25 worms are generally asymptomatic, and those with greater than 500 worms are considered severe. Red blood cell measures are useful for quantifying degree of anemia.

TREATMENT AND PREVENTION

Hookworm is easily treated with albendazole, mebendazole, or pyrantel pamoate. Demonstration that single-dose albendazole has good efficacy helped tremendously with mass deworming campaigns.

Child education in schools should focus on the value of foot coverings in endemic regions, proper hygiene, and nutrition. As is the case with all geohelminths, use of latrines greatly reduces the likelihood of transmission. Vaccine production efforts are underway. The identification of ancylostoma-secreted proteins (ASPs) has represented an important step in this process, and an ASP-derived vaccine is currently undergoing human testing.

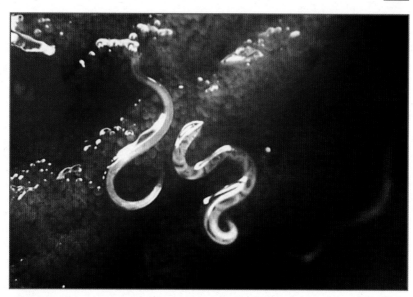

IMAGE 1

Hookworms are geohelminths. They live in soil and infect humans without the need for intermediate hosts or vectors. *Courtesy: Centers for Disease Control and Prevention.*

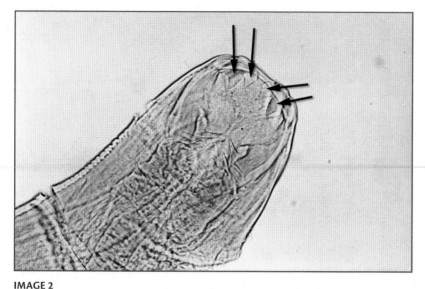

IMAGE 2

Adult *Ancylostoma* worms possess 4 hooklike teeth (depicted here). *Necator* species worms are armed with pairs of dorsal and ventral cutting plates. *Courtesy: Centers for Disease Control and Prevention/Mae Melvin.*

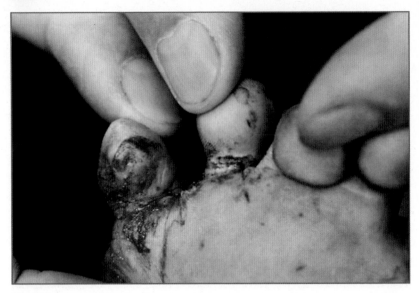

IMAGE 3
Ground itch may be the first sign of infection. Local dermatitis and itching occur at the site of larval penetration. *Courtesy: Centers for Disease Control and Prevention.*

Ascariasis

COMMON NAME

Giant intestinal roundworm

BACKGROUND

Ascariasis is caused by the parasitic nematode *Ascaris lumbricoides*. Humans are the sole host and, with up to 1.5 billion affected, ascariasis is the commonest helminthic infection worldwide. Poor environmental hygiene is the critical factor promoting disease, particularly in tropical regions and areas where human feces are used as fertilizer. Children aged 3 to 8 years are at greatest risk.

PATHOPHYSIOLOGY

Infection occurs via ingestion of fertilized eggs, primarily in food or water contaminated by fecal matter. Larvae hatch in the host's gastrointestinal tract, burrow through the small intestinal wall, and migrate passively in blood and lymph to the lungs. Following a 1- to 2-week maturation period, larvae penetrate alveolar walls, ascend the bronchial tree to the pharynx, and are swallowed. Mature larvae find their way to the small intestine but this time remain anchored to mucosal folds, actively swimming against the flow of chyme while they grow and develop into adult worms. By 2 months, females begin laying eggs and are remarkably productive: up to 200,000 ova can be excreted in stools each day. Following 1 to 4 weeks of soil incubation, ova become infective and lie in wait, potentially for years, to start the cycle anew.

CLINICAL PRESENTATION

Most patients remain asymptomatic, but clinically significant disease can occur during both larval and adult worm stages.

Ascaris pneumonitis develops during larval migration through the respiratory tract and is characterized by transient (approximately 10 days) fever, dyspnea, cough, and wheeze. When associated with eosinophilia, the term *Löffler syndrome* is applied.

Symptoms stemming from adult worms, when manifest, most commonly take the form of nonspecific dyspepsia, irritability, fatigue, and vomiting or diarrhea.

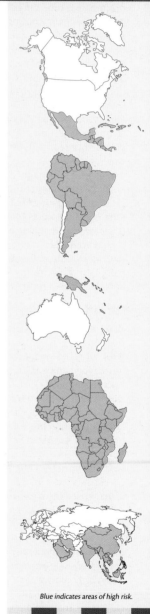

Blue indicates areas of high risk.

Adult worms may be noted incidentally in stools or exit through the mouth or nose. Migration from intestines can occur at any time but is found with greater frequency during times of stress, such as fever, anesthetic use, or antihelmintic treatment. Nomadic worms can be responsible for clogging biliary and pancreatic ducts, or invading the peritoneum. *Ascaris* adults are quite sizeable (up to 12 inches or 30 cm long) and live as long as 2 years. It comes as no surprise, then, that significant disease burdens can result in entangled worm masses that obstruct or perforate gut, especially in young children with small-caliber bowels. Adult worms feed on undigested intestinal contents rather than consume host blood; therefore, (1) anemia is uncharacteristic and (2) macronutrient and micronutrient deficiencies are not uncommon, principally in those suffering from a preexisting state of food insecurity.

DIAGNOSIS

Ascaris pneumonitis is a clinical diagnosis in endemic areas among children with suggestive respiratory symptomatology and eosinophilia. Sputum microscopy may reveal larvae, and transient pulmonary infiltrates are sometimes visible by radiograph. Because larval migration precedes egg production in the *Ascaris* life cycle, stool evaluation is negative during the pulmonary disease of primary infection.

Established adult worm infection is diagnosed through visualization of ova by stool microscopy. Given the tremendous numbers of eggs normally released by female worms, one specimen generally suffices (but beware false-negative evaluations when only male worms are present). *Ascaris* eggs are identified by a typical coarse, mammilated, albuminous coating. Abdominal radiographs and gastrointestinal contrast studies may demonstrate small intestinal filling defects, and worms can also be detected by ultrasonography. Be on the lookout for concomitant infection with other intestinal parasites.

TREATMENT AND PREVENTION

Pulmonary disease resolves spontaneously and antihelmintics are generally not administered during this stage, especially because larval death at this time may exacerbate symptoms. Steroids and bronchodilators may be of use in severe cases. Aggressive screening and treatment several weeks after respiratory illness, by which time worms will have matured and started shedding eggs, is recommended by some.

Traditional pharmaceutical regimens targeting *A lumbricoides* in children older than 2 years are mebendazole or single-dose albendazole. Single-dose pyrantel pamoate is an alternative. A test-of-cure stool examination can be performed 3 weeks following treatment but is not critical if symptoms improve.

Should intestinal obstruction complicate the clinical picture, initial management centers on bowel rest, intravenous fluids, and nasogastric tube bowel decompression; antihelmintics should be withheld until after the obstruction has resolved. Some children with intestinal, biliary, or other complications will require endoscopic or surgical intervention.

Enlightened preventive strategies combine chemotherapeutic regimens with improvement in sanitation services and health education. Because prevalence and morbidity are high in countries where ascariasis is endemic, many national health policies call for periodic (eg, every 3–6 months) mass empiric deworming of schoolchildren and others at high risk.

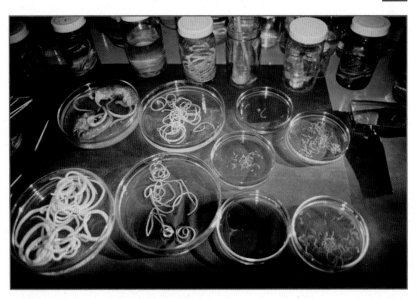

IMAGE 1
An unsettling laboratory collection in Peru. *Helminth* refers to an intestinal worm parasite, of which there are several varieties including nematodes (roundworms), cestodes (tapeworms), and trematodes (flatworms). *Courtesy: Kirsten Johnson.*

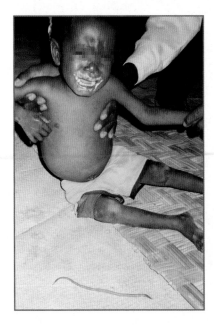

IMAGE 2
An adult worm, stressed by antihelmintic chemotherapy 2 days prior, found its way from the small intestine to the oral cavity and was expelled.

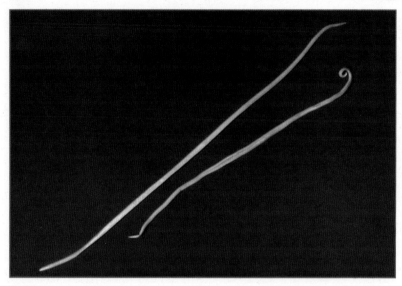

IMAGE 3

Adult *Ascaris* worms are cream-colored. Fully developed females are longer and distinguished by a darkened genital girdle band. Male worms, such as the smaller specimen depicted here, have a curved posterior end. *Courtesy: Centers for Disease Control and Prevention.*

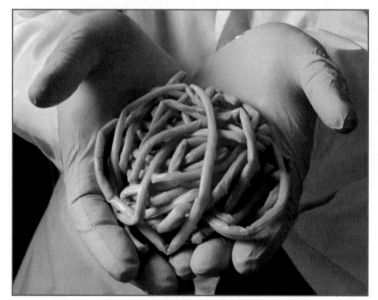

IMAGE 4

Worm burdens can be enormous within individual patients. This ascaritic mass was passed by a Kenyan child. *Courtesy: Centers for Disease Control and Prevention/Henry Bishop.*

Beriberi

COMMON NAMES

Ceylon sickness, Kakke, Loempe, Shoshin, Wernicke-Korsakoff syndrome

BACKGROUND

Beriberi is a disease of thiamine, or vitamin B_1, deficiency that chiefly affects the cardiovascular and nervous systems. Prevalence is highest in Southeast Asia and other countries where the diet staple is polished white rice, from which the thiamine-containing husk has been removed. Diets based heavily on degerminated maize meal, white flour, and cassava are also severely lacking in thiamine. Breastfed infants of thiamine-deficient mothers are at risk of beriberi, as are alcoholics and patients with underlying illness that impairs thiamine absorption. The condition also develops in displaced or imprisoned populations where nutrition access is limited and food variety is poor. Beriberi derives its name from the Singhalese (northeast Indian) phrase for "I cannot, I cannot," purportedly mimicking the cry of those incapacitated by the illness.

The most substantial sources of thiamine are cereals, vegetables, fruits, eggs, and milk. Heat, pasteurization, and other food processing procedures can destroy the vitamin.

PATHOPHYSIOLOGY

Thiamine diphosphate is a cofactor in carbohydrate metabolism and acetylcholine synthesis, which are processes essential to energy production, tissue maintenance, and integrity of the nervous system. Cardiovascular effects of beriberi stem from the weakening of myocardium and vascular smooth muscle. Direct neuronal injury and impaired nerve conduction result in nervous dysfunction. Other muscle layers throughout the body, including that of the gastrointestinal tract, are also damaged and contribute to widespread pain and debilitation.

CLINICAL PRESENTATION

Several forms of beriberi exist and are classified according to the affected body system. *Wet beriberi* describes patients suffering from cardiac illness and *dry beriberi* refers to those with primary neuritic involvement. Both

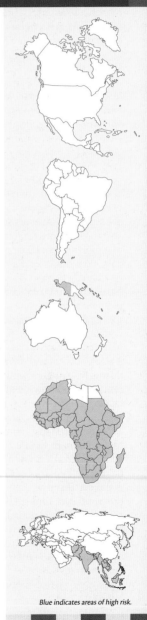

Blue indicates areas of high risk.

types frequently occur simultaneously, with one form predominating.

Wet beriberi is characteristically more acute at onset. Patients develop tachycardia, peripheral edema, and congestive heart failure. Older children appear pale with waxy skin and are frequently dyspneic. Fever, other evidence of sepsis, and structural cardiac disease are conspicuously absent. Dry beriberi often materializes insidiously with fatigue, irritability, anorexia, and weakness. With continued thiamine deficiency, progressive muscle wasting, polyneuritis, and peripheral neuropathy occur. Older children are pale and listless, and complain of paresthesias. Deep tendon reflexes of the lower extremities are reduced or absent. Symptoms referable to gastrointestinal tract involvement include constipation, abdominal pain, vomiting, and diarrhea.

Infantile beriberi develops in breastfed infants of thiamine-deficient mothers. Pallor, fussiness, and failure to thrive occur in the first several months. Cardiac failure can be abrupt. Babies may demonstrate an aphonic cry as a result of vocal cord paralysis. Older infants may present with symptoms resembling aseptic meningitis. Case-fatality rates in infantile disease are high.

Shoshin (translated from Japanese as "sudden collapse") is an uncommon fulminant variant of wet beriberi characterized by acute cardiovascular failure, pulmonary edema, and severe metabolic disturbances. Wernicke-Korsakoff syndrome denotes signs and symptoms attributable to cerebral beriberi and is observed mainly in alcoholics who suffer from a genetic abnormality in the thiamine-dependent enzyme transketolase.

DIAGNOSIS

A presumptive diagnosis is possible in at-risk populations when a diet history and clinical features are suggestive. Field case definitions usually incorporate signs including bilateral lower limb edema, dyspnea, paresthesias, and motor deficiencies. While laboratory resources for beriberi are often restricted in endemic areas, biochemical measurement of erythrocyte transketolase (a thiamine-requiring enzyme) activity is possible and can provide a useful functional assessment of thiamine reserves. The thiamine pyrophosphate effect, a direct assay for transketolase, is elevated in beriberi and may be helpful. Urinary thiamine excretion can also be measured, usually over 24 hours, or over 4 hours following a test dose of thiamine. Nonspecific electrocardiogram findings in wet beriberi are prolonged QT interval, T wave inversion, and low voltage. In many settings, a clinical response to thiamine treatment is the most practical means by which to confirm thiamine deficiency.

TREATMENT AND PREVENTION

Beriberi is treated with thiamine supplementation. Oral administration is preferred but intramuscular or intravenous formulations are used in severe cases. The body naturally excretes excess thiamine, so overdoses and adverse effects are rare. Children with wet beriberi typically exhibit a dramatic clinical response to therapy within hours. Electrocardiogram changes can quickly revert to normal. The peripheral neuropathy that characterizes dry beriberi takes longer to heal—improvement occurs gradually over several months. Physical therapy during treatment is beneficial. Other potential nutritional deficiencies should be aggressively identified and treated.

In endemic countries, educational campaigns help to teach families why beriberi develops and how to prevent it. Ensuring consumption of a balanced diet constitutes the critical intervention. Recommended daily dietary intake of thiamine increases with age and ranges from 0.3 to 1.2 mg. Requirements are increased in pregnant and lactating women. Vitamin supplements may be available and advisable for some children.

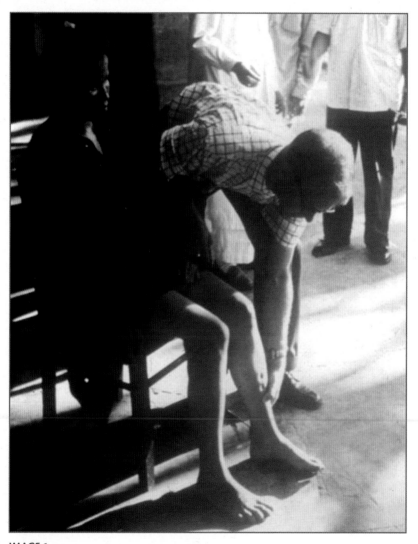

IMAGE 1

Pitting edema is demonstrated in a woman from the Orient who suffers from the cardiovascular effects of wet beriberi. *Courtesy: Centers for Disease Control and Prevention.*

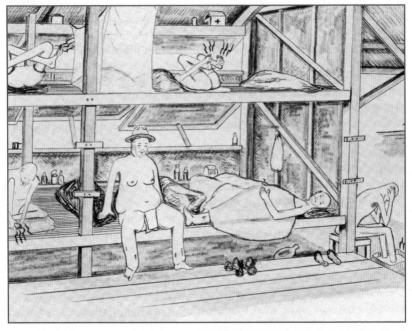

IMAGE 2

A 1942 sketch depicting attitudes of wet and dry beriberi during World War II. Beriberi was noted when troops in the Philippines were restricted to quarter rations. Prisoners of war also demonstrated typical clinical features. Debility, muscle wasting, pedal edema, pain, and paresthesias are evident in the drawing. At the time, disease was treated with massive doses of thiamine administered intraspinally (not currently recommended) and intramuscularly. *Courtesy: Office of Medical History, Office of the Surgeon General, United States Army.*

Burkitt Lymphoma

BACKGROUND

Burkitt lymphoma (BL) is an aggressive, high-grade, non-Hodgkin B-cell malignancy found predominantly in equatorial Africa. The tumor is named for Denis Burkitt, a surgeon who described the lesion in Uganda in the 1950s while working with His Majesty's Colonial Service. Male children are most commonly affected, usually near the end of the first decade of life. Endemic, sporadic, and immunodeficiency-related forms of BL exist and are distinguished by their geographic location, involved body compartments, and risk factors. Burkitt lymphoma accounts for more than 30% of childhood lymphomas worldwide and 75% of all malignancies in endemic areas. Endemic disease, which primarily affects the jaw, is found in damp regions of Papua New Guinea and the so-called Burkitt belt, a swath of central Africa stretching between 10 degrees north and south of the equator. Endemic BL is highly linked with Epstein-Barr virus (EBV) (the EBV genome is incorporated into most Burkitt lymphomas) and possibly malaria. Sporadic BL occurs outside of Africa and Papua New Guinea. It is morphologically similar to the endemic form but chiefly occupies the abdominal viscera, targets a broader age range, and is coupled with EBV in a minority of cases. Immunodeficiency-related disease develops in the context of HIV/AIDS and is responsible for most adult cases of BL.

PATHOPHYSIOLOGY

All forms of BL are histologically similar and are associated with molecular translocations involving chromosome 8 that deregulate the *c-myc* oncogene. Translocations between chromosomes 8 and 14 are observed most frequently, followed by those involving chromosome 8 and chromosome 2 or 22. Monoclonal proliferation of B lymphocytes occurs at an extremely rapid clip, and BL is among the fastest-growing malignancies. Cell doubling time is 1 to 2 days.

CLINICAL PRESENTATION

Early, nonspecific constitutional symptoms include weakness, anorexia, weight loss, night sweats, and fevers. Rapidly growing malignant infiltration of the mandible

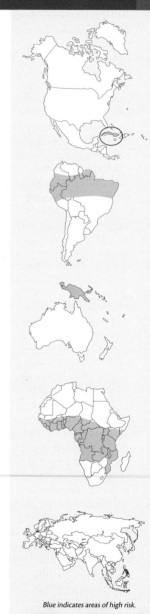

Blue indicates areas of high risk.

and maxilla is the principal finding in endemic BL. Children present with jaw pain, soft tissue swelling, and loose teeth. Lymphadenopathy is possible but not universal. Metastasis to the bone marrow, meninges, gonads, and kidneys follows. Sporadic BL typically involves abdominal organs, particularly the ileocecal intestinal tract or stomach. The kidneys, breast, ovaries, and thyroid may also be affected, and tumor is known to metastasize to bone marrow, lymph nodes, and the nervous system. Abdominal distension with ascites and associated pain is a common presentation of sporadic BL. Bowel obstruction or gastrointestinal bleeding may also develop.

Four stages of BL are recognized that range from a single, non-mediastinal, non-abdominal extranodal tumor (stage I) to widespread, multi-organ disease with bone marrow or central nervous system (CNS) involvement (stage IV).

DIAGNOSIS

Diagnosis of BL in many resource-limited settings relies on clinical suspicion combined with histopathologic examination of a fine-needle aspirate or biopsy of involved tissue. The microscopic appearance of a Burkitt tumor at low power assumes a "starry sky" appearance created by light-colored macrophages containing apoptotic cell debris scattered over the dark, dense background of malignant lymphoid cells. Burkitt cells are monomorphic and medium-sized with round nuclei and basophilic cytoplasm. Features of tumor lysis, including elevated serum lactate dehydrogenase and uric acid, may be present. Cytogenetic analysis or fluorescent in situ hybridization can reveal characteristic translocations. Additional investigations including bone marrow biopsy, cerebrospinal fluid evaluation, radiography, computed tomography, or bone scan may be useful for assessing the spread and stage of disease.

TREATMENT AND PREVENTION

Systemic chemotherapy is the mainstay of therapy and can be effective even in advanced cases. Endemic BL often responds to a protocol consisting of cyclophosphamide, vincristine, and prednisone administered weekly for 3 weeks then monthly for an additional 3 courses. Monotherapy with cyclophosphamide may also be effective. Methotrexate can be valuable for CNS disease and for CNS prophylaxis. Cytarabine and doxorubicin are other commonly used agents. Monoclonal antibodies are used in selected protocols in conjunction with chemotherapy. Intravenous hydration before and during chemotherapy is important to prevent complications from tumor lysis syndrome.

In optimal circumstances, cure rates approach 60% to 80% in disseminated disease and 90% in localized disease. Unfortunately, these relatively high cure rates may not be realized in low-income regions due to later presentation of disease and the fact that the mass appears clinically resolved after the first round of chemotherapy. Many times children do not return for the final rounds of chemotherapy until the tumor is again clinically evident. With immunodeficiency-related BL, chemotherapy is poorly tolerated and the prognosis is generally poor.

Few proven preventive measures against BL are recognized. Improving local health care systems to ensure early diagnosis and referral is vital to maximizing the effect of chemotherapy. Decreasing the incidence of malaria may be beneficial because of its implication as a possible cofactor in BL. Similarly, protection against HIV will reduce BL related to immunodeficiency.

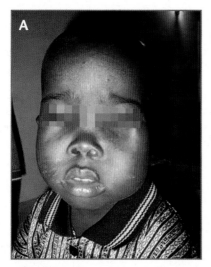
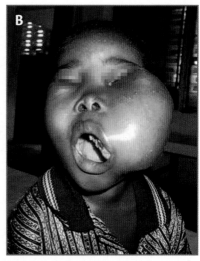

IMAGE 1A, 1B

An 11-year-old Liberian child presented with a jaw mass of several months' duration. Transfer was arranged to a hospital, a day's drive away, with capacity for treating Burkitt lymphoma. The family never arrived at the referral center and, instead, had elected to seek treatment from a local traditional healer. Six weeks later, the mass was considerably larger. Liberia is located in the Burkitt belt of sub-Saharan Africa. *Courtesy: Andrew Schechtman.*

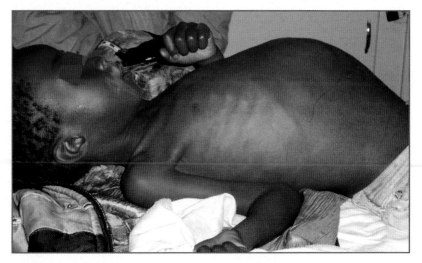

IMAGE 2

A previously well Zambian boy was noted by his father to have abdominal swelling 2 weeks before presentation. The mass was easily palpated and extended across the entire abdomen. Abdominal Burkitt lymphoma was diagnosed. Shortly after the first round of chemotherapy, the tumor was no longer palpable. *Courtesy: Charles J. Schubert.*

Burns

BACKGROUND

Burns occur frequently in the tropics, particularly in children younger than 4 years, and can result in devastating long-term consequences. Most burns are caused by hot liquid. Other causes of burn injury include radiation, radioactivity, friction, electricity, and chemical substances. Flame burns often stem from ignition of highly flammable, loose cotton clothing. Chemical burns result from acids or other corrosive materials to which children are exposed by direct contact or accidental consumption. Intentional burns inflicted by traditional practices have been reported. Burns may also be associated with celebratory events (eg, fireworks injury during festivals).

Most burns take place in homes, especially at sites of food preparation. As such, burns most frequently occur in the late morning period and during evening mealtime when food is prepared, cooked, and served. Overall incidence is greater among boys, although young girls who assist with kitchen chores are also at high risk. Poor socioeconomics increases the likelihood of burns by negatively affecting housing conditions, child supervision, and types and location of heating sources.

PATHOPHYSIOLOGY

Heat-induced burn severity depends on both the temperature and duration of exposure. Thermal energy inflicted in a quantity or rate that exceeds the body's ability to dissipate heat leads to cell injury and subsequent necrosis of skin and underlying tissues. The primary processes involved in burn wound healing—epithelialization, contraction, and scar formation—may be functionally impaired in children who live in poor communities as a result of inadequate nutrition, poor hygiene, and chronic or secondary infection. Keloid formation, a possible complication of burn wound healing, seems to be more common in dark-skinned individuals.

CLINICAL PRESENTATION

Presentation of burned children may be delayed due to transport challenges or a preference for traditional

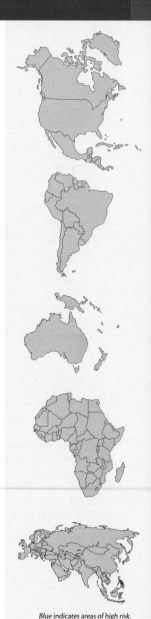

Blue indicates areas of high risk.

treatments. Comprehensive wound assessment includes the depth, extent, and specific location of burns. First degree, superficial burns involve the epidermis only and are characterized by pain and erythema without blisters. As a rule, first degree burns are not included when determining the percentage of body surface area involved. Second degree, or partial-thickness, burns extend to the dermis and are painful, pink or red, moist, and blistering. Third degree, full-thickness burns involve the entire dermis and are pale, white, black, or yellow-brown in color. Blistering is absent and, because nerve endings are damaged, lesions are painless. Fourth degree burns are uncommon and extend through subcutaneous tissue to bone, joint, or muscle. They result many times from high-voltage electrical injury. Burns to the face, hands, feet, joint folds, and perineum are more severe because of the functional limitations they impose. Patient age and underlying health conditions are important to note, as is the risk of potential associated injury (eg, smoke or toxic gas inhalation).

DIAGNOSIS

Unintentional burns pose no diagnostic problems in the context of a complete history and physical examination. Burns involving unusual body compartments or lesions that are inconsistent with presenting histories represent important clues to distinguish between accidental and inflicted burns.

TREATMENT AND PREVENTION

Basic first-aid treatment including topical antiseptic (eg, gentian violet) is sometimes applied by local caretakers prior to presentation. Mild and moderate burns should be gently washed with soap and cool, clean water. Ice is contraindicated. Blisters are best left intact to minimize the risk of infection. Application of silver sulfadiazine or other antimicrobial ointment is often recommended. Cleansed wounds should be covered with sterile gauze. Dressings should be changed regularly.

Severe burns predispose to hypovolemic shock through large insensible losses and increased capillary permeability. Vascular access and fluid resuscitation are critical components of care in these children. Respiratory compromise can result from smoke inhalation (causing hypoxia, airway mucosal edema, or carbon monoxide poisoning), pneumonia, or impaired chest wall compliance from circumferential full-thickness burns. Local wound care is essential. Dead tissue should be removed, lesions cleansed, and local antimicrobial paste applied. Fevers may only constitute a response to large burns, and systemic antibiotics are not administered unless infection is suspected. Tetanus prophylaxis, nutritional care, and early physiotherapy are important treatment adjuncts. Pain management is a vital consideration in all burn patients. Analgesics are frequently used, especially during debridement and dressing changes. Whenever possible, children with substantial burns should be transported to a formal burn unit. Skin grafting may be necessary.

Childhood burns in the tropics are largely preventable. At the family level, interventions focus on environmental modifications, parental education, proper storage of flammable or otherwise toxic substances, and adequate child supervision. Broader solutions address socioeconomic conditions and product design (eg, inexpensive, safe kerosene stoves).

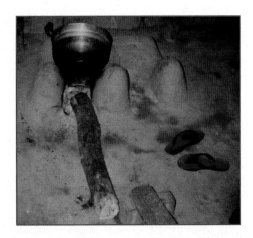

IMAGE 1

Indoor stoves are found in many homes worldwide. The tripod firestone depicted here is made of dried mud or earth and fueled by lighted firewood that sits at ground level. The apparatus is within easy reach of children. *Courtesy: Samuel N. Forjuoh.*

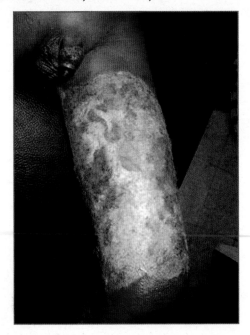

IMAGE 2

Two weeks prior to presentation, this child was scalded by a pot of hot water that tipped from a cooking fire. The filamentous growth on his well-healing burn was not identified until the mother stated that she had applied animal fur, a common traditional remedy in her village. *Courtesy: Andrew Schechtman.*

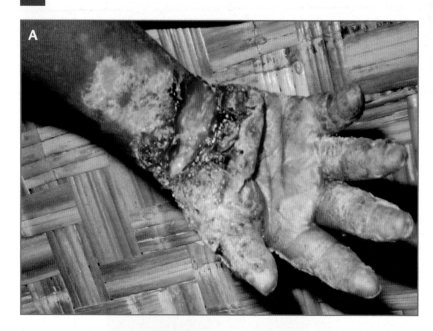

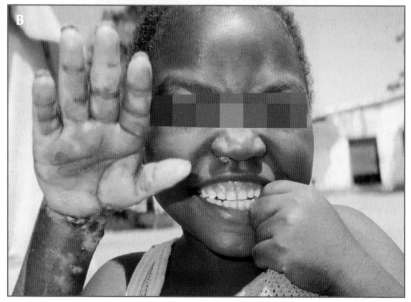

IMAGE 3A, 3B

A second- and third-degree burn to the wrist and hand healed extremely well with meticulous local care. The importance of early and consistent physical therapy cannot be overstated in patients with joint wounds.

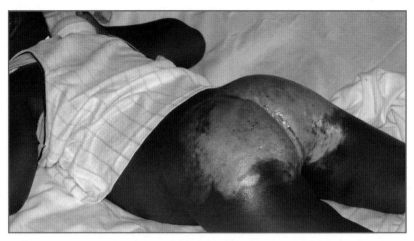

IMAGE 4

A young boy reportedly sustained extensive burns to the buttocks and perineum by falling in a saucepan that contained hot cooking oil. Caregivers must reconcile mechanism of injury with physical findings and fully protect children by ruling out abuse. *Courtesy: Samuel N. Forjuoh.*

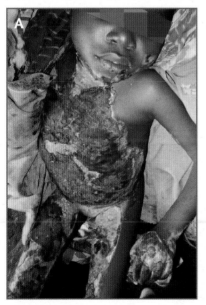
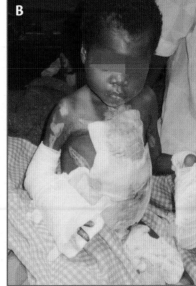

IMAGE 5A, 5B

Extensive flame burns to this patient's trunk and limbs resulted when her clothing caught fire from a nearby open flame. This type of severe burn is at high risk for complication by hypovolemic shock and airway compromise. Pain management is essential. There exists just cause for optimism, even for significant injuries. This hopeful, strong-willed girl survived and was a source of inspiration for all who worked with her.

Buruli Ulcer

BACKGROUND

Buruli ulcer is a chronic, necrotic soft tissue lesion caused by *Mycobacterium ulcerans*. The condition takes its name from Buruli County, Uganda, where some of the first cases were described in the 1960s. Prevalence is highest in sub-Saharan and West Africa, but endemic foci also exist in the Americas, Asia, and the Western Pacific. Children younger than 15 years are at greatest risk. The precise mechanism through which transmission of *M ulcerans* occurs is unclear, although associations are likely with antecedent trauma and nearby water bodies.

PATHOPHYSIOLOGY

Minor skin injuries probably abet inoculation of *M ulcerans*, which subsequently proliferates in sub-cutaneous fatty tissue and secretes a destructive toxin called *mycolactone*. Local necrosis leads to the develop-ment of characteristic ulcers. Mycobacteria can spread to contiguous muscle or bone, and can metastasize via blood or lymph. In early stages, the toxin asserts an immunosuppressive effect that facilitates ulceration. Over time, host immunity strengthens. Healing begins with accumulation of an inflammatory exudate, fol-lowed by epithelialization and granuloma formation.

CLINICAL PRESENTATION

Non-ulcerated cutaneous findings precede skin break-down and take the form of painless papules, nodules, or adherent plaques. The extremities, predominantly the lower limbs, are involved in 90 % of cases. Lesions evolve over a period of weeks to months, necrosing centrally to form a wide ulcer with distinctive undermined edges. Multiple ulcers can communicate under overlying skin and, therefore, scope of affliction may be worse than it appears. Invasion of joints and bone can be particularly deforming. Patients are typically pain-free and afebrile, which delays presentation. A rapidly progressive form of disease is characterized by diffuse, non-pitting, pain-less edema that extends rapidly and forms a large ulcer. Most wounds eventually heal spontaneously. Primary morbidities are cosmetic disfigurement and permanent physical disabilities resulting from the healing process. Twenty-five percent of children suffer debilitating scars, contractures, ankylosis, or lymphedema.

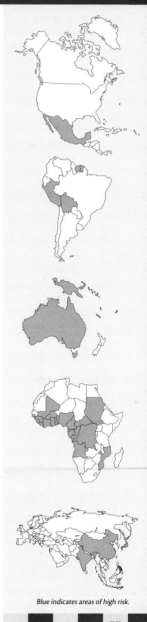

Blue indicates areas of high risk.

DIAGNOSIS

Tissue smears obtained from ulcer edges can be stained to reveal acid-fast bacilli, although sensitivity is low because mycobacterium load is nominal within lesions and distribution of organisms is not uniform. While *M ulcerans* is slow-growing, culture on Löwenstein-Jensen agar is possible. Histopathology is technically more involved but highly sensitive. Coagulation necrosis of subcutaneous adipose tissue in the presence of extracellular acid-fast bacilli is a distinguishing feature. When available, testing by polymerase chain reaction is effective and rapid.

TREATMENT AND PREVENTION

Combination antibiotic therapy with rifampicin and streptomycin is the preferred first-line treatment for most patients with Buruli ulcer. With therapy, recurrence rates are relatively low. Wide surgical excision of necrotic tissue was standard of care for many years, but surgery is now generally reserved for debridement, skin grafting when necessary, and management of refractory cases. Physical therapy is essential to both treat and prevent contractures, especially in young children.

While no vaccine specific to Buruli ulcer is available, it has been suggested that bacille Calmette-Guérin immunization may ameliorate disease. Recommendations for disease prevention in endemic regions include promoting feet and leg covering, maintaining good hygiene of traumatic wounds, and using protected wells to reduce contact with potentially contaminated environmental water sources.

Buruli ulcer is a classic "neglected" disease that primarily affects rural populations in underdeveloped countries. These groups possess little market or policy influence to encourage research and development of new therapies. In 1998 the World Health Organization launched the Global Buruli Initiative to help coordinate efforts of research communities, health ministries, nongovernmental organizations, and donors. This effort is ongoing.

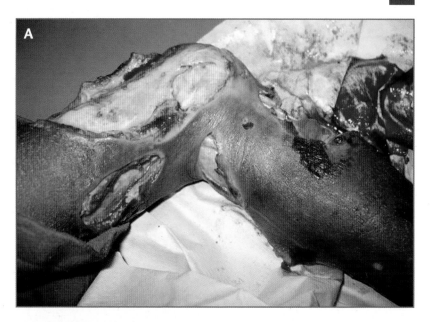

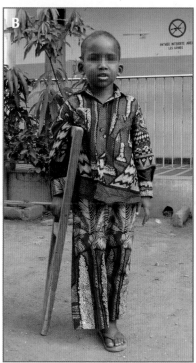

IMAGE 1A, 1B

A 10-year-old boy in Cote D'Ivoire presented with extensive painless ulcers of 6 months' duration on his lower leg. Civil conflict and financial constraints had precluded earlier care seeking. The image shows the wounds following only minor debridement. Some improvement was noted following several weeks of parenteral antibiotics but, sadly, amputation was eventually felt to represent the most humane option given the extent of damage and deformity that had occurred. This case was extreme; amputation is rarely necessary for Buruli ulcer. *Courtesy: Keri Cohn.*

Carrion Disease

COMMON NAMES

Oroya fever, Peruvian wart disease, verruga peruana

BACKGROUND

Carrion disease is a 2-staged illness caused by the intra-cellular gram-negative *Bartonella bacilliformis*. Disease occurs in the inter-Andean valleys of Peru, Colombia, and Ecuador, especially between 2,000 and 8,000 feet above sea level where the insect vector thrives. Prevalence in endemic regions can be as high as 15%. Individuals younger than 20 years are most affected.

PATHOPHYSIOLOGY

The female hematophagous sandfly, *Lutzomyia verrucarum*, is the vector responsible for transmission. Following the insect's bite and an incubation period that ranges 10 to 210 days (mean incubation is 2 months), disease manifests in 2 consecutive stages. The first stage, Oroya fever, is acute at onset and cor-related with bacteremia. Hemolysis can lead to severe anemia, and endothelial cell damage risks microvascu-lar thrombosis. Both processes contribute to end-organ ischemia. Mortality rates are high in untreated patients. Those who survive the first phase of illness enter a second stage 2 weeks to 2 years later, which involves a skin eruption known as *verruga peruana*.

CLINICAL PRESENTATION

Oroya fever can develop insidiously with a brief, non-specific febrile illness that is poorly recognized. These mild cases account for patients who subsequently develop verruga peruana but deny having had the first stage of illness. Alternatively, Oroya fever may pres-ent fulminantly, with prolonged fever, anorexia, and arthralgias. Pallor and jaundice result from hemolysis, and mental status deterioration and shock can ensue. Generalized lymphadenopathy and hepatosplenom-egaly are common. A transient cellular immunosup-pression follows in 30% of patients and predisposes to superinfections, including invasive salmonella or reactivated tuberculosis or toxoplasmosis.

The appearance of verruga peruana can be diverse. Miliary forms are intensely erythematous,

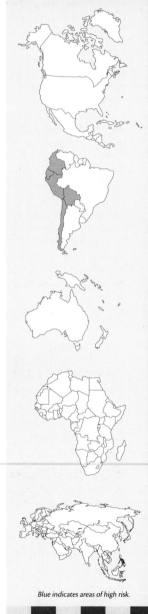

Blue indicates areas of high risk.

angiomatous, circular papules measuring 1 to 4 mm that resemble hemangiomas. They are more common on the lower extremities and are often pruritic. Subcutaneous nodules may also appear. These are larger than miliary lesions and do not alter overlying skin. Finally, so-called mulaire lesions are possible and characterized by protruding blood-filled papules measuring greater than 5 mm that ulcerate and bleed easily. Systemic symptoms may be present but are less common during this second stage of disease.

DIAGNOSIS

A high index of suspicion in endemic areas is essential. Anemia, hyperbilirubinemia, and transaminitis occur frequently. Intra-erythrocytic organisms can be identified on thin smear in most patients with Oroya fever, and *B bacilliformis* can be cultured from blood. Serologic testing is available but is not widely used. During the eruptive phase, definitive clinical diagnosis requires demonstration of characteristic histopathologic changes on skin biopsy including proliferation of capillaries, endothelial cells, monocytes, and macrophages. Warthin-Starry tissue stain permits bacteria identification.

TREATMENT AND PREVENTION

Aggressive antibiotic therapy in the Oroya fever stage significantly decreases mortality. Ciprofloxacin is the preferred treatment and chloramphenicol, in combination with ampicillin, is an effective alternative. Blood transfusions may be necessary during this phase. Azithromycin is first-line therapy for verruga peruana. Rifampin is also effective, but in certain settings concern exists regarding resistance development, particularly for multidrug-resistant tuberculosis. Preventive strategies focus on encouraging behaviors that guard against insect vector bites.

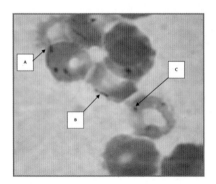

IMAGE 1

A Giemsa-stained blood smear demonstrates coccobacillus (A), bacillus (B), and coccus (C) forms of *Bartonella bacilliformis*. *Courtesy: Palmira Ventocilla.*

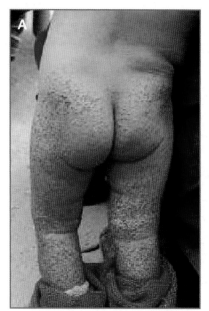 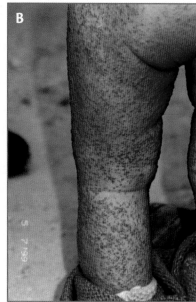

IMAGE 2A, 2B

A preschool child is afflicted with the cutaneous miliary form of eruptive Peruvian wart disease. Note the pantslike distribution affecting the legs and buttocks. *Courtesy: Ciro Maguiña.*

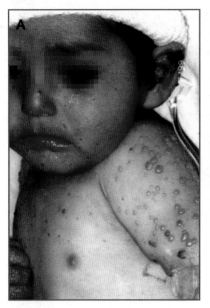
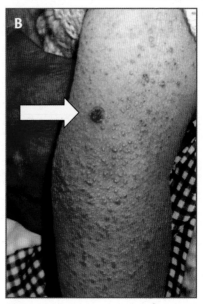

IMAGE 3A, 3B
An atypical form of verruga peruana can be similar in appearance to chickenpox and is sometimes referred to as a verrucous or pseudo-varicella form of illness. However, lesions here are larger than are seen with varicella and rupture less easily. Both miliary and mulaire (arrow) type lesions are evident. *Courtesy: Ciro Maguiña.*

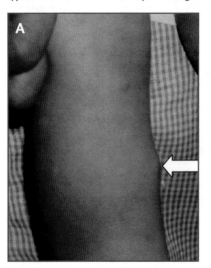
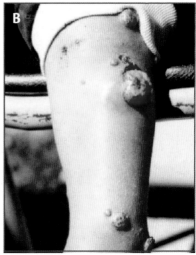

IMAGE 4A, 4B
Subcutaneous Peruvian wart disease in a toddler (Image 4A, arrow) and bacillary angiomatosis due to *Bartonella bacilliformis* (Image 4B). *Courtesy: Ciro Maguiña.*

Chikungunya Fever

BACKGROUND

Chikungunya fever is a reemerging viral disease caused by chikungunya virus (CHIKV), an RNA virus belonging to the family *Togaviridae* and genus *Alphavirus*. The disease is almost always self-limiting and is rarely fatal. Molecular characterization has demonstrated 2 distinct strain lineages that cause epidemics in Africa and Asia. These geographical genotypes exhibit differences in transmission cycles: a sylvatic cycle in Africa is maintained between monkeys and wild mosquitoes while in Asia the cycle exists between humans and *Aedes aegypti* mosquitoes. In 2005 an outbreak occurred on the French islands of La Reunion, Mayotee, Mauritius, and Seychelles. In the same year, CHIKV reappeared in India after nearly 3 decades of quiescence, with 1.3 million suspected cases in 12 states.

PATHOPHYSIOLOGY

Chikungunya virus is most commonly transmitted to humans through the bite of infected *Aedes* mosquitoes, although vertical transmission is also possible. High viremia is typical during the first 2 days of illness, declines at days 3 and 4, and usually disappears by day 5. "Silent" CHIKV infections may occur in children. Chikungunya virus infection, clinically evident or silent, is thought to confer lifelong immunity.

CLINICAL FEATURES

Incubation following mosquito bites averages 48 hours but may be as long as 12 days. Symptom onset is abrupt and heralded by fever and severe arthralgia, followed by constitutional symptoms and rash lasting for a period of 1 to 7 days. Fever rise can be dramatic, often reaching high temperatures and accompanied by intermittent shaking chills. Arthralgias are polyarticular and migratory, and predominantly affect the small joints of hands, wrists, ankles, and feet, with lesser involvement of larger joints. Patients in the acute stage may complain bitterly of pain when asked to ambulate and they characteristically lie still. Joint swelling may occur, but fluid accumulation is uncommon. Mild articular manifestations usually resolve within a few weeks, but more severe cases may remain symptomatic for months.

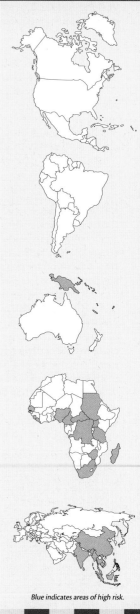

Blue indicates areas of high risk.

Generalized myalgias, back pain, and shoulder discomfort are common.

Cutaneous manifestations begin with flushing over the face and trunk and evolve to an erythematous dermatitis. The trunk and limbs are most frequently involved, but lesions may also appear over the face, palms, and soles. The rash eventually simply fades or desquamates.

Infection can infrequently result in meningoencephalitis, particularly in newborns and those with preexisting medical conditions. Chikungunya outbreaks typically result in several hundreds or thousands of cases, but deaths are rare.

DIAGNOSIS

Chikungunya fever should be suspected when epidemic disease occurs with the characteristic triad of fever, rash, and rheumatic symptoms. Virus-specific IgM antibodies can be helpful with diagnosis. Chikungunya virus isolation from blood is accomplished by either in vivo (mice or mosquito) or in vitro techniques. Chikungunya virus detection is also possible in early stages using traditional polymerase chain reaction (PCR) methods. A specific and sensitive 1-step PCR assay has recently been developed as a rapid indicator of active infection by quantifying viral load in clinical samples or cell culture supernatant.

TREATMENT AND PREVENTION

Chikungunya fever is usually self-limiting, and no specific treatment exists. Rest and supportive care are indicated during acute joint symptoms. Movement and mild exercise tend to improve stiffness and morning arthralgia, but heavy exercise may exacerbate rheumatic symptoms. Nonsteroidal anti-inflammatory drugs may be beneficial, and chloroquine has been used in severe cases. Infective persons should be protected from mosquito exposure so that they do not contribute to further transmission.

No vaccine is available, and preventive efforts are focused on vector control. Elimination of breeding sites or source reduction is important. Larvivorous fish (eg, gambusia, guppy), which eat mosquito larvae, may be introduced into local endemic areas. Protection from mosquito bites is achieved by insect repellent and use of insecticide-treated mosquito nets, especially during the daytime when the mosquitoes feed. Well-planned fogging operations are sometimes recommended in high-risk villages, where clustering of cases has been reported. Active epidemiological surveillance for CHIKV is crucial for promoting effective community education and transmission control.

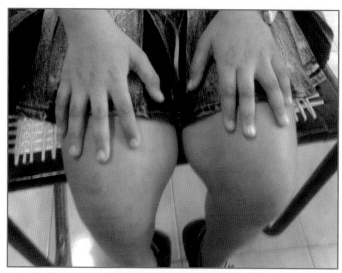

IMAGE 1

Joint swelling is typical of Chikungunya infection. Knees and small joints of the hands may be affected. *Courtesy: Mala Chhabra, Veena Mittal and Shiv Lal.*

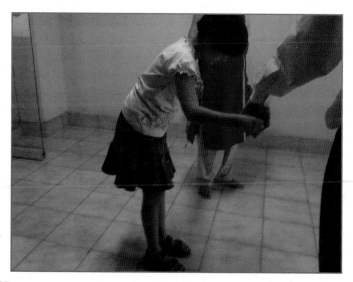

IMAGE 2

The Makonde ethnic group inhabits parts of Mozambique and Tanzania. Chikungunya fever derives its name from the Makonde word meaning "that which bends up," in reference to the arthritic posture assumed by those severely affected. The image depicts an affected girl in India who has chikungunya-related joint pain. *Courtesy: Mala Chhabra, Veena Mittal and Shiv Lal.*

Cholera

COMMON NAMES

Asiatic cholera, rice-water diarrhea

BACKGROUND

Vibrio cholerae is the etiologic agent of cholera, a diarrheal illness that commands particular respect for its ability to cause rapid, potentially fatal dehydration. While more than 100 serogroups cause disease, *V cholerae* O1 (globally) and O139 Bengal (Southeast Asia) are most important because they can give rise to explosive epidemics.

Cholera is endemic in Asia, Africa, Southern Europe, and Central and South America. The organism is believed to have originated near the Ganges Delta, stretching over India and Bangladesh, an area affected since at least the time recorded history began. Seven worldwide pandemics have been recognized since the early 1800s, the last starting in Indonesia (1961), subsequently spreading to Africa (1971) and the Americas (1991), and persisting to present day. Cholera is a reportable condition to the World Health Organization (WHO) and has an annual global burden that exceeds 1 million people.

Motile vibrios can live free in aquatic reservoirs. Humans are the only known host, and transmission is fecal-oral. Ingestion of contaminated water and food is the commonest mode of infection.

States of overcrowding and poor sanitation as exists, for example, in camps of displaced persons create a dangerously perfect milieu for cholera outbreaks. In endemic regions, attack rates are highest among children aged 1 to 4, in whom acquired immunity is less well developed. Once ingested, gastric acidity represents one of the body's few defense mechanisms; as such, individuals with *Helicobacter pylori* gastritis and hypochlorhydria, and those taking antacids or histamine blockers, are also at increased risk.

PATHOPHYSIOLOGY

V cholerae is a gram-negative, comma- or S-shaped slender bacillus. Organisms multiply rapidly in the alkaline environment of the proximal small intestine and elaborate a potent enterotoxin. Cholera toxin

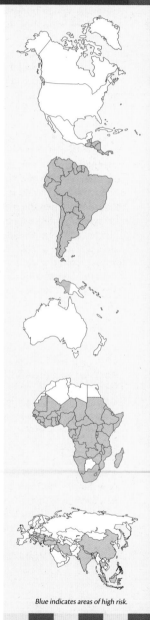

Blue indicates areas of high risk.

65

consists of 2 fragments: the B subunit clings to local enterocytes and facilitates intracellular entry of the A subunit, which upregulates cyclic adenosine monophosphate production triggering copious ion and water efflux. A dramatic secretory diarrhea results, with substantial loss of sodium, potassium, and bicarbonate. Despite the outpouring of fluid, inflammation is minimal and the intestinal epithelium remains remarkably intact.

CLINICAL PRESENTATION

Fortunately, most patients remain asymptomatic. When disease manifests, the incubation period is 1 to 5 days. Mild-to-moderate diarrhea may be the extent of illness. Less than 5% of infected children develop the startling clinical picture of cholera gravis: acute, profuse, painless watery diarrhea accompanied by emesis and severe dehydration. Children are at risk for hypoglycemia. Fever is uncommon. Spasmodic abdominal pain and muscle cramping are possible. Metabolic acidosis, hypovolemic shock, renal failure, altered mental status, coma, and death can occur within hours. Mortality rates in untreated patients approach 50%. For those who survive, cholera is self-limiting, and diarrhea resolves in a week or so.

DIAGNOSIS

Isolation of vibrios is generally more important for defining an outbreak than for managing individual cases. *V cholerae* growth on selective media, usually thiosulphate citrate bile salt sucrose agar, remains the diagnostic gold standard. Organisms can also be identified by dark-field examination of a stool wet preparation. Direct antigen detection dipstick tests are now available and, because results are available in minutes, can be extremely useful.

When dipstick diagnoses are made, samples should also be formally tested at a reference laboratory for confirmation and determination of antimicrobial sensitivities.

TREATMENT AND PREVENTION

The mainstay of treatment is rapid and sustained rehydration. With appropriate therapy, case-fatality rates should be less than 1%.

Oral rehydration solution (ORS) is effective and represents the preferred first-line treatment for children who are minimally dehydrated. Quantity administered should match stool and emetic output. In resource-limited settings, ORS also can be used to manage patients suffering from moderate dehydration who are able to drink. Oral rehydration solution can be infused via nasogastric tube when necessary. Use of newer rice-based or amylase-resistant starch ORS formulations is advocated by some.

Rapid and aggressive intravenous fluid replacement is indicated for restoration of blood volume in children who are more than moderately dehydrated or who are shocky. Lactated Ringer's is the solution of choice. Normal saline is an alternative as long as ORS is added quickly to supplement base and potassium. Fluid administration rates must be closely monitored in infants and severely malnourished children, who are at risk of cardiac overload.

Antibiotics eradicate vibrios and reduce illness duration and severity. A 3- to 5-day course is advisable for patients who are more than mildly ill. Erythromycin is frequently used, but antimicrobial sensitivities should guide treatment whenever possible. Potential alternatives include doxycycline, ciprofloxacin, azithromycin, trimethoprim-sulfamethoxazole, and tetracycline. Adjunctive zinc has been shown to lessen stool output. Antimotility agents, adsorbents, analgesics, and antiemetics are not recommended.

Cholera prevention efforts are centered on improving systems that promote quality sanitation, provide safe water, and ensure good food hygiene. Antimicrobial prophylaxis has a limited role, although administration within 24 hours of index case identification may prevent transmission to close contacts. In the event of outbreaks, timely public health interventions are essential for limiting spread. Several cholera vaccines exist, all with limited efficacy. That said, the WHO states that oral cholera vaccine may be suitable for travelers and may also have a role in selected complex emergencies.

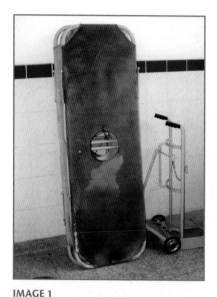

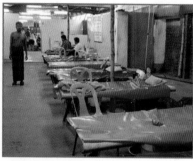

IMAGE 2

A row of cholera cots at a cholera hospital in Bangladesh. Measuring fluid quantities collected in buckets is important for determining fluid balance. With proper rehydration, recovery can be dramatic. *Courtesy: Robert de Leeuw.*

IMAGE 1

A cholera cot represents quintessential appropriate technology. Patients lie supine with their rear over the hole, and a bucket below. Cholera gravis is frequently so debilitating, with such frequent stools, that traditional use of a toilet or pit latrine is impossible.

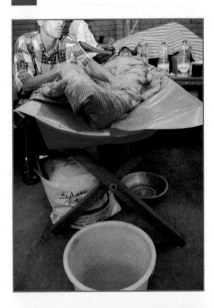

IMAGE 3

Diarrhea in cholera is watery with mucous flecks, so-called rice-water stool. *Courtesy: Robert de Leeuw.*

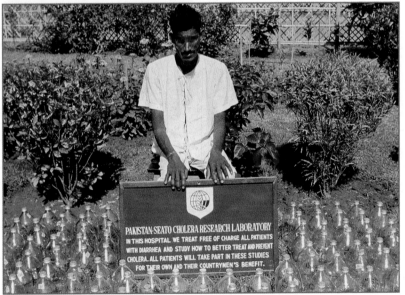

IMAGE 4

As a young physician working in Bangladesh, Dr Richard Cash was instrumental in completing the first successful clinical trial of oral rehydration therapy on patients with severe diarrhea. He captured this image of a cholera survivor who required nearly 100 liters of fluid resuscitation. The gentleman is sitting amidst all of the 1-L intravenous fluid bottles, now empty, that were required during his treatment. *Courtesy: Richard Cash.*

Cutaneous Larva Migrans

COMMON NAMES

Creeping eruption, ground itch, sandworms

BACKGROUND

Cutaneous larva migrans is distributed worldwide but chiefly affects children living in the tropics and subtropics. It is also a common, albeit unwelcome, souvenir dermatosis brought home by travelers returning from beach holidays in Southeast Asia, the Caribbean, Central and South America, and the Southeastern United States. Filariform larvae of the animal hookworm *Ancylostoma braziliense* are the most frequent culprits, although other parasitic nematodes have also been implicated.

PATHOPHYSIOLOGY

Adult *Ancylostoma* hookworms live attached to mucosa in the gastrointestinal tract of dogs and cats, and shed their eggs with host feces. Ova hatch in sand or soil and release larvae, which molt and become infective. In the parasite's natural life cycle, larvae penetrate fur and skin of a new animal host, migrate via venous and lymphatic channels to the lungs, breach the alveoli, climb the bronchial tree, and are swallowed. They mature in the intestinal cavity to adulthood and begin the cycle anew.

Humans are accidental hosts. Exposure to contaminated sand or soil, such as occurs when walking barefoot or sunbathing, permits larval infiltration of the superficial layers of intact human skin. However, unlike in animal hosts, larvae lack the ability to pierce the epidermal basement membrane in humans and thus have no access to other organ systems. Instead, larvae are trapped in the epidermis, where they amble haphazardly for the remainder of their short life and produce the serpiginous burrows that are the hallmark of the disease.

CLINICAL PRESENTATION

Children may recall a stinging sensation, which occurs sometimes as larvae penetrate skin. The rash begins as an itchy red papule and progresses to a pruritic, erythematous, elevated, curvilinear skin eruption.

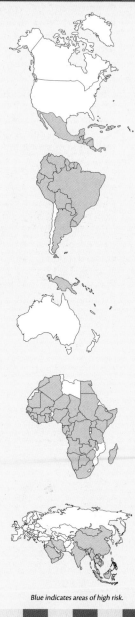

Blue indicates areas of high risk.

The migrating track, generally 2- to 4-mm wide, corresponds to the advancing edge of wandering larvae and can extend up to 1 to 2 cm daily. The distal lower extremities are most frequently affected, but lesions can involve any exposed skin surface, including the thighs, buttocks, chest, and hands. Pruritis is often severe; reactive scratching can be so vigorous as to bring about secondary bacterial infection. Lesions resolve after larvae die (within a period of weeks to months), with complete resolution of symptoms even in those who are untreated.

DIAGNOSIS

Diagnosis is clinical and based on pertinent history in the setting of characteristic skin burrows. Returning travelers who are affected often note having enjoyed themselves in the sun and sand at a tropical location, and may remember seeing stray dogs or cats in the area. Peripheral eosinophilia and elevated serum IgE levels may be present, but laboratory evaluation is not required. Biopsy is not recommended.

TREATMENT AND PREVENTION

While the condition is self-limited, intense pruritis and risk for secondary infection generally mandate treatment. Oral albendazole is the agent of choice. Pruritus resolves within 1 to 3 days, and serpiginous tracts clear a week later. Ivermectin and thiabendazole are effective alternatives. Antihistamines and topical steroids can be used in conjunction with antihelmintics for symptomatic relief. Antibiotics are indicated for secondary bacterial complications. Prevention is accomplished by avoiding direct skin contact with contaminated surfaces (eg, by use of footwear or beach towels when spending time on sand in high-risk areas). Sandboxes or beaches should be protected from potentially infected animals, which should also be periodically dewormed.

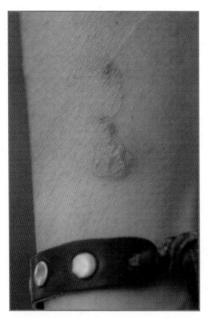

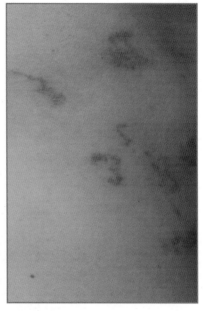

IMAGE 1

Humans are "dead-end" hosts for animal hookworms, but unfortunately the parasite is oblivious to this fact! The elevated, serpiginous lesion seen here can cause a relentless itch and be aesthetically unpleasant. *Courtesy: Gorgas Memorial Institute of Tropical and Preventive Medicine.*

IMAGE 2

When infective larvae are given the opportunity to invade at numerous sites, multiple tracts can develop. Treatment is straightforward. *Courtesy: Gorgas Memorial Institute of Tropical and Preventive Medicine.*

Cysticercosis

BACKGROUND

Cysticercosis is caused by the cestode *Taenia solium*. This pork tapeworm is globally dispersed, but disease is rarely found in countries that benefit from well-regulated meat industries. Central and South America, parts of Africa, and Southeast Asia are most affected. *T solium* is the commonest parasitic infection involving the central nervous system and represents a major cause of epilepsy in less developed settings. Approximately 50 million people worldwide harbor the organism.

PATHOGENESIS

To understand clearly the pathogenesis of cysticercosis, one must also be familiar with a related *T solium* illness, human taeniasis.

Ingestion by children of *T solium* larval cysts (cysticerci) in undercooked pork leads to taeniasis, a tapeworm infection. Worms mature to hermaphroditic adults, each composed of hundreds of 5- to 10-mm proglottid segments, and attach themselves via hooklets and suckers to the small intestine mucosa. Adult tapeworms can live for years in the gastrointestinal tract, and they shed gravid segments, packed with eggs, into the environment each day. In the tapeworm's "normal" life cycle, pigs consume eggs in food sullied by human feces. Eggshells are digested in swines' stomachs and release oncospheres that enter the bloodstream and find their way to muscle, where cysts form. In this cycle, *T solium* exploits 2 species: pig (the intermediate host) and human (the definitive host).

Human cysticercosis is a more serious illness that develops when children ingest eggs (rather than cysticerci) and "accidentally" host the intermediate form of *T solium*. This sometimes occurs by autoinfection. Oncospheres released from eggshells penetrate the intestinal mucosa and disseminate to distant sites. A tropism exists for neural, ophthalmologic, muscle, hepatic, and subcutaneous tissues. Cysticerci, sometimes referred to as *bladder worms,* are transiently characterized by a worm head and body before transforming into a transparent vesicle with clear fluid that measures up to a centimeter in diameter. Disease

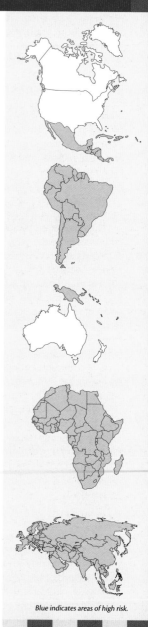

Blue indicates areas of high risk.

severity is related to cyst burden, tissue types affected, and intensity of host immune responses. Much of the morbidity associated with cysticercosis stems from brain and spinal cord involvement, so-called neurocysticercosis. Clinical "flares" spurred by immune reactions can happen years after the initial infection, when cysts begin to die.

CLINICAL PRESENTATION

Intestinal tapeworm disease may be asymptomatic or result in nonspecific anorexia, nausea, and abdominal pain. Proglottid segments may be visualized in the stool. Rarely, worm migration to other body compartments leads to more esoteric symptoms.

The incubation period for cysticercosis varies widely, usually between 6 months and 5 years. Focal seizures in a previously healthy child are a frequent clinical manifestation and the reason most patients present. Secondary generalization of fits is possible. Elevated intracranial pressure may develop either from obstructive hydrocephalus or cerebral edema caused by multiple brain cysts (a condition known as *cysticercotic encephalitis*). Spinal cord involvement can produce motor disturbances. Other complications include chronic headache and mental status changes.

Subcutaneous nodules (generally painless and moveable) and visual impairment result from cysticerci lodging in soft tissue and the eye, respectively.

DIAGNOSIS

Taeniasis is diagnosed by identification of proglottids or eggs in feces. Diagnosis of cysticercosis is fairly straightforward in many regions of the world when epidemiological, clinical, and radiologic data are combined. Computed tomography or magnetic resonance imaging demonstrating cystic lesions with circumferential inflammation and edema is highly suggestive. Neuroimaging is important to define number and location of lesions because this is relevant to management of neurocysticercosis. Cerebrospinal fluid characteristics are not specific, and lumbar puncture should not be performed in children with evidence of raised intracranial pressure. Subretinal parasites may be seen on funduscopic examination. Serology is available but has limited sensitivity and specificity. Enzyme-linked immunoelectrotransfer blot (Western blot) assay is more reliable.

TREATMENT AND PREVENTION

Praziquantel is often used to treat tapeworm infection. Anticonvulsants are standard in the management of neurocysticercosis, but antiparasitic use is controversial. Host immunity may be able to contain infections with few brain cysticerci. When numerous cysts are present, treatment can elicit an intense and dangerous inflammatory response as parasites die. Uniform recommendations are impossible. Treatment should be individualized and care plans established in collaboration with local experts.

If administered, cestidal therapy is usually with albendazole or praziquantel. Patients should be hospitalized and first given corticosteroids to both lessen cerebral edema associated with cysts and prophylactically minimize immune reactions that are expected from dying cysticerci. Surgical intervention may be required for management of hydrocephalus or spinal cysticercosis unresponsive to medical treatment.

Good hygiene and adequately cooking pork are the most effective mechanisms for breaking the *T solium* transmission cycle. Individuals with suspected tapeworm infection should be treated immediately.

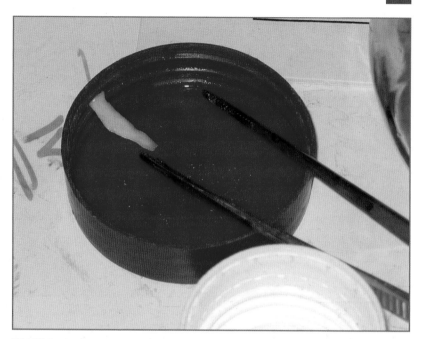

IMAGE 1

Adult *Taenia solium* worms can grow to near 4 m in length. The head (scolex) is globular with 4 suckers and a double row of hooklets. Hundreds, potentially even a thousand, proglottid segments are typical. Shown is one segment, identified in human feces, of what is sure to be a much larger worm.

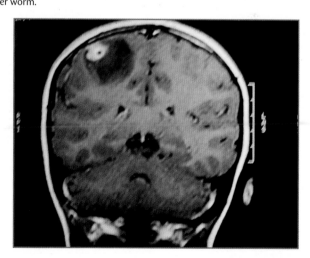

IMAGE 2

Computed tomography reveals the classic brain lesion in a patient with neurocysticercosis. *Courtesy: Ashok Kapse.*

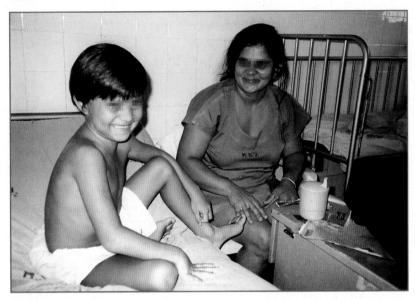

IMAGE 3

A young boy in northern Brazil appears well but presented with focal seizures from neurocysticercosis. He is receiving anticonvulsants. The decision to provide antiparasitic therapy was made, and he was admitted to the hospital for corticosteroids and monitoring during treatment.

Dengue

COMMON NAME

Breakbone fever

BACKGROUND

Dengue is a potentially fatal viral illness transmitted through the bite of infective *Aedes* mosquitoes, most commonly *Aedes aegypti*. Four distinct serotypes of dengue virus are recognized and belong to the genus *Flavivurus*, a family that also contains the agents responsible for tick-borne and Japanese encephalitides. Several clinical dengue syndromes exist, including dengue fever, dengue hemorrhagic fever, and dengue shock syndrome. Disease develops sporadically or in epidemics in Southeast Asia, Africa, the Pacific, and tropical Central and South America. Heavily populated urban areas are at particularly high risk. Worldwide, more than 50 million cases of dengue fever and several hundred thousand cases of dengue hemorrhagic fever occur each year. More than 2 billion people live in dengue-endemic parts of the world.

PATHOPHYSIOLOGY

Adult *A aegypti* mosquitoes tend to seek human blood meals during daytime, when streets are crowded, and commonly feed on multiple individuals during a single meal. Children acquire dengue through the bite of an infected mosquito and, when they subsequently develop febrile viremia, become the source through which naive mosquitoes contract the virus. Infection confers lifelong immunity to the infecting serotype, but susceptibility remains to disease from other serotypes. All serotypes produce similar disease.

Dengue hemorrhagic fever and shock syndrome are thought to occur in children who previously had dengue fever and were then later exposed to a different dengue serotype. These conditions are therefore rarely seen in travelers but rather affect children living in endemic regions who have a higher likelihood of repeated infections. Reexposure seems to trigger an antibody complex response that results in vascular damage, intravascular fluid leak, and bleeding.

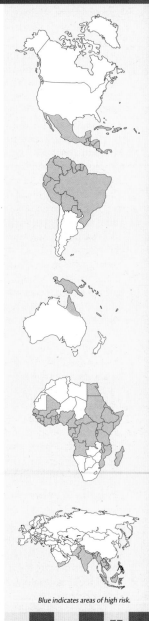

Blue indicates areas of high risk.

CLINICAL PRESENTATION

Dengue Fever

The spectrum of disease ranges from mild to severe. In endemic regions, dengue may manifest clinically only as a nonspecific viral illness. Others become very ill. Following an incubation period of 3 to 8 days, children present with symptoms including sudden onset of high fever, coryza, malaise, headache, retro-orbital discomfort, nausea, and anorexia. Many children also report a change in taste sensation. Lymphadenopathy occurs regularly. Dengue facies syndrome is characterized by swollen eyelids and conjunctival injection. Severe muscle, joint, and body pains can develop and have earned the nickname *breakbone fever*. Rash develops in half of patients and appears as scarlatiniform, maculopapular, or morbilliform. Areas of erythema can be occasionally interspersed with patches of normal skin. Mild evidence of bleeding may exist by way of petechiae and gingival bleeding. Defervescence happens after several days, but then recurs in half of patients—a biphasic temperature pattern referred to as *saddleback fever*. Disease generally resolves by the seventh day, but weakness, malaise, and anorexia may persist for weeks. Fortunately, dengue fever in children is usually a self-limited disease without significant complications.

Dengue Hemorrhagic Fever

Dengue hemorrhagic fever is a more serious illness primarily affecting children and adolescents native to endemic regions. The acute phase resembles dengue fever, but considerable bleeding develops near the time of defervescence.

Hemorrhage occurs in the skin (eg, petechiae, ecchymoses, purpura), mucous membranes (eg, gingival bleeding, epistaxis), and gastrointestinal tract (eg, hematemesis, melena). Circumoral or peripheral cyanosis may follow. Oozing from venipuncture sites is common.

Dengue Shock Syndrome

Progression to circulatory failure results from increased capillary permeability and intravascular leak. Hypotension, pleural effusions, and generalized edema develop. The pulse turns thready. Patients become pale and restless or lethargic. Severe abdominal pain, wide swings in body temperature, and mental status changes are additional harbingers of frank shock and possible fatality.

Dengue hemorrhagic fever and shock syndrome are classified by the World Health Organization as grade I (fever, nonspecific symptoms, mild hemorrhagic signs), II (spontaneous bleeding), III (circulatory failure), and IV (profound shock).

DIAGNOSIS

Diagnosis is frequently made on clinical grounds. Leukopenia and thrombocytopenia are common. Hematoconcentration often results in elevation of the hematocrit to more than 20% above baseline. Relative bradycardia despite fever is sometimes observed. Bleeding propensity is assessed by the "tourniquet test," positive when 20 or more petechiae per 2.5 cm^2 arise after a sphygmomanometer on the upper arm is inflated to a point midway between the systolic and diastolic pressures for 5 minutes. Definitive laboratory diagnosis is achieved by serology or direct isolation of virus from serum.

TREATMENT AND PREVENTION

Management of dengue fever is focused on symptomatic relief and treatment or prevention of dehydration. Acetaminophen (paracetamol) is standard. Aspirin, which has anti-clotting effects, is not to be used. During epidemics, a high index of suspicion for hemorrhagic fever and shock syndrome is critical because, without treatment, mortality rates exceed 20%. Young children and those with evidence of shock, bleeding, or severe thrombocytopenia should be hospitalized. The most critical intervention is restoration of intravascular volume, with normal saline or lactated Ringer's. Packed red blood cell and fresh frozen plasma transfusion is recommended to treat extensive bleeding. Hemodynamic instability, orthostasis, or persistent hypotension despite fluid resuscitation may necessitate ionotropic support. Intramuscular injections are contraindicated.

Beneficial behavior change strategies for prevention include increasing coverage with mosquito nets and insect repellent. Poorly planned urbanization promotes disease by creating vector breeding sites. Conversely, community-wide education programs that encourage the removal of standing water sources can reduce dengue outbreaks.

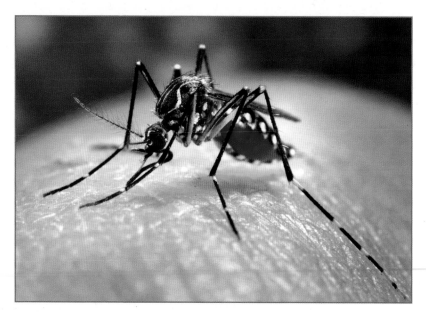

IMAGE 1

Aedes aegypti mosquitoes typically lay eggs in artificial containers that collect water in urban, poverty-stricken settings (eg, discarded automobile tires, buckets, and trash barrels). *Courtesy: Centers for Disease Control and Prevention/Frank Collins, Center for Global Health & Infectious Diseases, University of Notre Dame.*

Diphtheria

BACKGROUND

Diphtheria is an acute toxin-mediated disease caused by *Corynebacterium diphtheriae* that primarily affects the tonsils, pharynx, nose, and skin. Signs and symptoms depend on the site of infection, the immunization status of the host, and whether exotoxin has been systemically distributed. In 2002 the World Health Organization estimated 5,000 deaths from diphtheria, of which nearly 4,000 occurred among children younger than 5 years. Crowding and poor personal hygiene contribute to transmission of diphtheria bacilli. Four biotypes of *C diphtheriae* can be distinguished on biochemical testing: *gravis*, *mitis*, *intermedius,* and *belfanti*. Recently, most infections have been caused by *gravis* or *mitis* biotypes. Sucrose-fermenting *C diphtheriae,* a biotype uncommonly seen in industrialized countries, has been associated with diphtheria outbreaks and cases of endocarditis in developing countries.

PATHOPHYSIOLOGY

Diphtheria toxin, which kills sensitive cells by blocking protein synthesis, is a 58 kDa polypeptide consisting of fragment A, which has enzymatic activity, and fragment B, which participates in binding of and entry into host cells. Toxigenic *C diphtheriae* infection on the mucosal surface results in the formation of a characteristic pseudomembrane. Edema and hyperemia of the infected surface are followed by necrosis of the epithelium, accompanied by outpouring of a fibrinosuppurative exudate. Severe lesions have marked vascular congestion, interstitial edema, fibrin exudation, bacterial cells, and intense neutrophil infiltration. Diphtheria toxin passes into the bloodstream and can affect all cells in the body, but most prominently the heart, producing myocarditis; the kidney, resulting in renal tubular necrosis; and the nervous system, resulting in demyelination.

CLINICAL PRESENTATION

Faucial diphtheria involves the posterior structures of the mouth and proximal pharynx. The onset is usually slow, with low-grade fever, anorexia, malaise, sore throat, nausea, vomiting, and painful dysphagia. The earliest pharyngeal finding is generally mild

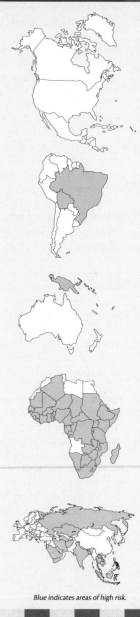

Blue indicates areas of high risk.

81

erythema. A characteristic patch or patches develop of a grayish or white adherent membrane with a surrounding dull red inflammatory zone on one or both tonsils that bleeds with scraping. Later in the course of infection, the membrane may have areas of green or black necrosis, the lymph nodes in the neck are enlarged and painful, and the neck may be slightly swollen. Secretions of affected tissue emanate a fetid odor.

Nasal diphtheria, usually mild and often chronic, is marked by seropuru- lent or serosanguineous nasal discharge that can incite erosion of the external nares and upper lip.

Laryngeal and tracheobronchial diphtheria may result from extension of a pharyngeal infection or represent pri- mary infection sites. Moderate fever and gradually increasing hoarseness, stridor, and cough are typical. Obstruction of breathing by the expanding pseudomembrane and associated edema is possible and occurs progressively over about 24 hours. Respiratory embarrass- ment, severe adenitis, and soft tissue edema result in a "bull neck" appear- ance in advanced cases. The severely affected individual appears agitated, but is quiet, sweating, and ominously cyanotic. The use of accessory muscles of respiration is marked by retraction of supraclavicular, substernal, and inter- costal tissues on inspiration. Suffocation and death may result without urgent intervention (eg, tracheostomy).

A severe malignant form of diphthe- ria is acute in onset. Children become rapidly toxic, with high fever, tachy- cardia, hypotension, and cyanosis. Bleeding from the mouth, nose, and skin is possible. Cardiac involvement with heart block occurs early. More than 50% of malignant cases are fatal, and this high mortality rate changes little with treatment. Erasure edema

of the neck may also be noted in completely immunized individuals.

Common sites for cutaneous diphtheric lesions are the lower legs, feet, and hands. An ulcerative lesion known as *ecthyma diphtheriticum* is the presenting lesion, which is painful and may be covered with an adherent dark pseudomembrane during the first 1 to 2 weeks. Concomitant nasopharyngeal infection occurs in 20% to 40% of patients.

Unusual sites of infection include the buccal mucosa, upper and lower lips, hard and soft palate, and tongue. *C diphtheriae* also has been isolated from conjunctiva, ears, esophagus, stomach, vagina, and sperm.

Myocarditis is an important toxic complication of diphtheria. Atrioventricular dissociation, complete heart block, and ventricular arrhythmias are associated with high mortality rates. Evidence of cardiac toxicity can appear as early as the first or as late as the sixth week of illness. The frequency of cardiac involvement following laryngeal and malignant diphtheria is also higher if antitoxin administration is delayed more than 48 hours after onset of disease.

Approximately three-fourths of patients with severe disease develop neuropathy. The incidence of neuro- logic complications is related directly to the severity of respiratory symp- toms. Neuropathy is first indicated by paralysis of the soft palate and poste- rior pharyngeal wall, often resulting in regurgitation of swallowed fluids through the nose. Thereafter, cranial neuropathies causing oculomotor and ciliary paralysis may produce blurred vision. Paralysis of the pharynx, larynx, and respiratory muscles are common.

Additional complications include submucosal or skin petechial hemor- rhages, acute tubular necrosis, arthritis, pericarditis, disseminated intravascular coagulation, and respiratory coinfections such as pneumonia or bronchitis.

DIAGNOSIS

Suspected, probable, and confirmed diphtheria cases should be immediately reported to health authorities. Diphtheria is no longer easily diagnosed on clinical grounds, particularly in those countries where the disease is rarely seen.

In its early stages, diphtheria may be mistaken for a severe viral pharyngitis. Both culture of *C diphtheriae* and a positive toxin-production assay are required for confirmation of the diagnosis. In cases of suspected respiratory diphtheria, samples obtained from the throat and nasopharynx should be cultured before initiating antibiotic treatment. If a membranous material is present, samples should be obtained from beneath its edge. Any wound or skin lesion should also be swabbed. A serum sample should be obtained before administration of antitoxin for measurement of antibodies to diphtheria toxin, as demonstration of a non-protective level may support the diagnosis if cultures are negative.

TREATMENT AND PREVENTION

Specific treatment should be provided under the direction of a consultant in infectious diseases. The occurrence of diphtheria requires immediate control measures, including treatment and isolation of the index case, and vaccination and chemoprophylaxis of contacts. During an outbreak, special measures such as mass immunization may be required.

If diphtheria is suspected, specific treatment with diphtheria antitoxin and antibiotics should be initiated without waiting for bacteriologic confirmation.

Antitoxin dose, ranging from 20,000 to 100,000 U intramuscularly or intravenously depends on the site, the degree of toxicity, and the duration of illness. Before antitoxin is administered, patients should be tested for sensitivity to horse serum and, if necessary, desensitized. Delayed administration increases the risk of late effects such as myocarditis, neuritis, and nephritis.

The antibiotics of choice are erythromycin, azithromycin, clarithromycin, or penicillin. Resistance to penicillin G and erythromycin has been documented. Children should be cared for in strict isolation until bacteriologic clearance has been demonstrated at least 24 hours after completing treatment.

Close contacts should be clinically assessed for symptoms and signs of diphtheria and kept under daily surveillance for 7 days from the date of the last contact with the case.

The recommended schedule for vaccination against diphtheria varies considerably between countries. In addition to childhood immunizations, populations living in low-endemic or non-endemic areas may require booster injections of diphtheria toxoid at 10-year intervals to ensure lifelong protection. Special attention should be paid to immunizing health care workers who may have occupational exposure to *C diphtheriae* and travelers to diphtheria-endemic countries. The need for booster doses in adults should be determined by serologic surveys.

Unfortunately, diphtheria infection does not always confer protective immunity. Individuals recovering from the disease should therefore complete active immunization with diphtheria toxoid during convalescence.

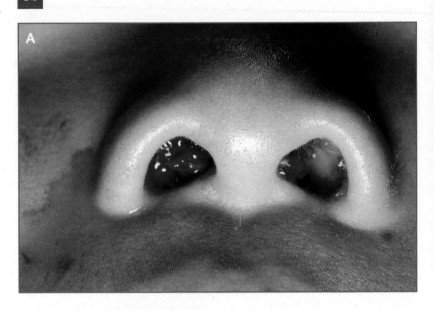

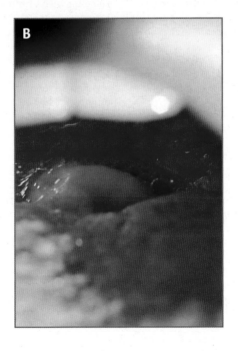

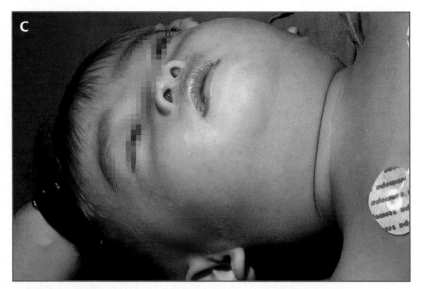

IMAGE 1A–1C

Diphtheria patients with nasal (Image 1A) and pharnygeal (Image 1B) membranes. The nose and pharynx should be examined carefully to identify these features in children who present with fever, nasal discharge, sore throat, and foul odor. Some children present with severe edema of the neck, known as *bull neck* (Image 1C). *Courtesy: Bryan Watt and Leila Srour.*

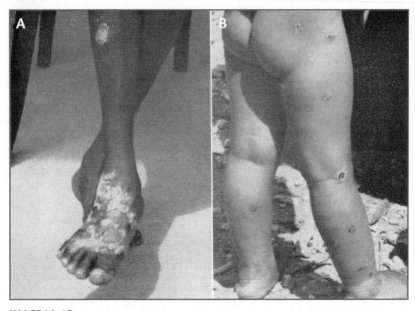

IMAGE 2A, 2B
Diphtheric skin lesions may manifest as open wounds. *Courtesy: Office of Medical History, US Office of the Surgeon General.*

Dracunculiasis

COMMON NAMES

Guinea worm, Medina worm, pharaoh worm

BACKGROUND

Dracunculiasis follows ingestion of freshwater contaminated with copepods (water fleas) that contain the parasitic nematode *Dracunculiasis medinensis*. The affliction is ancient. It has been identified in a 3,000-year-old mummy and is believed to be described in the Old Testament as the "fiery serpent" responsible for torturing the Hebrews during their exodus from Egypt. Mortality is generally low, but secondary bacterial infections may be life-threatening due to lack of access to health care in most endemic areas. Associated painful and infected ulcers can substantially impair mobility and incapacitate patients for weeks or months.

The presence of Guinea worm disease in a community usually indicates extreme poverty and the absence or inadequacy of safe drinking water. The health status and livelihoods of entire villages may be negatively affected if children are prevented from attending school and adults from tending their fields or livestock.

Once prevalent in 20 nations in Africa, the Middle East, and Asia, Guinea worm disease affected approximately 3.5 million people when eradication efforts began in 1986. The Global Dracunculiasis Eradication Campaign (led largely by The Carter Center, founded by former US President Jimmy Carter and his wife, Rosalynn) has dramatically reduced the number of cases to fewer than 5,000 reported in 2008. Only 6 endemic countries remain: Sudan, Ghana, Mali, Ethiopia, Nigeria, and Niger.

PATHOPHYSIOLOGY

Transmission occurs by accidental consumption of tiny *Cyclops* copepods, often found in stagnant pond water, that have ingested *D medinensis* larvae. Though stomach digestive juices kill the copepods, the larvae of the Guinea worm survive and penetrate the stomach or small intestinal wall, migrating to the subcutaneous tissue of the abdomen and thorax. During the next 2 to 3 months, these larvae develop into adult worms and mate. The male worms die shortly after copulation

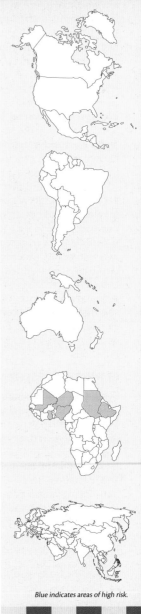

Blue indicates areas of high risk.

while females continue to mature and burrow into connective tissue and along long bones. Approximately a year following initial infection, female worms emerge through the dermal surface. Dependent regions including the foot and lower leg are the most common exit points, although any part of the body can be involved. Often multiple worms can appear at the same time—as many as 40 or more have been documented to emerge simultaneously. A blister forms at the site of egress, and the associated burning sensation elicited by worm penetration is relieved by soaking the affected limb.

Submerging the affected body part in water triggers gravid females to release hundreds of thousands of microscopic larvae, a particularly unfortunate occurrence when released in a community water source. These larvae are then ingested by copepods, completing the life cycle. There is no acquired immunity to Guinea worm, so simple prevention techniques such as water filtration and health education are required to avoid repeated infections.

CLINICAL PRESENTATION

Symptoms from migrating adult parasites are rare but may include an urticarial rash, fever, nausea, vomiting, diarrhea, and dizziness. Worms emerge over a period of weeks and produce intensely painful edema, blistering, and ulceration. Baseline health and nutritional status play important roles in determining the rate and success of ulcer healing. The process may be prolonged and, in many cases, is complicated by secondary bacterial infection, abscess formation, septic arthritis, sepsis, or tetanus. Joint infection may result in deformities and limb contractures. The mean length of disability is 10 weeks, although some patients experience continuing pain for an additional 12 to 18 months.

DIAGNOSIS

Guinea worms are diagnosed clinically as they approach dermal tissue and form a painful papule, which subsequently enlarges and ruptures to expose the adult worm. Immersion of affected body parts in water can lead to a characteristic "white cloud," representing release of larvae.

TREATMENT AND PREVENTION

At present, no medications are available to treat or prevent dracunculiasis. Pain is addressed symptomatically with analgesics, although these are rarely available in the remote areas where the disease remains endemic. Antibiotics are critical for management of superinfections. Affected limbs should be kept clean, disinfected, and bandaged. Emerging worms are easily torn if pulled with force. Instead, extrusion is facilitated by curling worms around a small stick and manually winding them several centimeters daily. This method, which is painful and can take up to a month, has been practiced for centuries. Some scholars suggest that this traditional treatment for Guinea worm is the basis for the caduceus and staff of the Aesculapius symbol of medicine.

Dracunculiasis eradication strategies are focused on behavior modification and health education. Nylon water filters or specially designed filtration straws effectively strain copepods. Affected individuals are encouraged not to soak their affected limbs in areas where water is used for public consumption. Vectors are targeted through treatment of water sources with the safe larvicide temephos and the construction of boreholes or deep wells.

A number of favorable disease features render Guinea worm a promising candidate for eradication: seasonality is marked, assisting the timing and effectiveness of surveillance and control interventions; human carrier states are limited to the 1-year incubation period and no animal reservoir exists; the intermediate host is contained (not mobile, such as mosquito vectors); the diagnosis is relatively easy and worm protrusion is required for transmission; and the methods for controlling transmission are not complex. The Global Dracunculiasis Eradication Campaign, working in partnership with endemic countries, hopes that disease elimination will be achieved within the next several years. Guinea worm will be the first parasitic disease to be eradicated in human history.

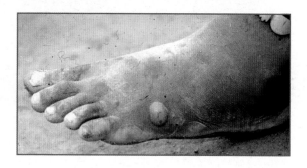

IMAGE 1

This tell-tale blister, which forms up to a year following infection, is the first sign of Guinea worm disease. During the next 24 to 48 hours, the blister will burst and the worm will emerge. Even though a burning sensation often results, patients should be instructed not to cool the wound by placing it in a community water source. *Courtesy: The Carter Center.*

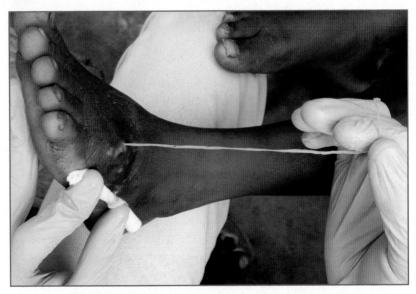

IMAGE 2

A threadlike, whitish guinea worm burns a hole from inside and breaks through the skin. Dracunculiasis derives its name from the Latin term for "affliction with little dragons." *Courtesy: The Carter Center/Louise Gubb.*

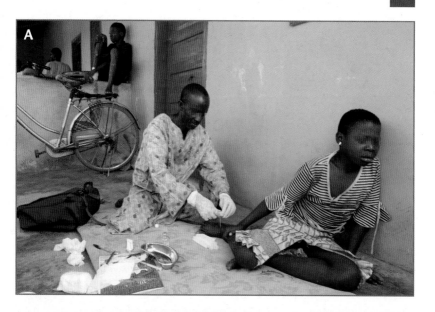

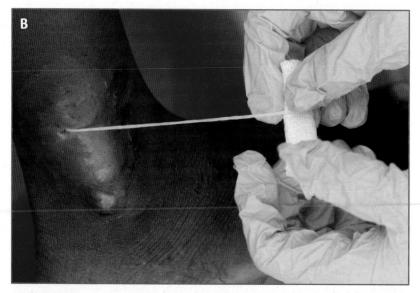

IMAGE 3A, 3B

A local health worker removes a guinea worm from the foot of a 9-year-old patient in Ghana (Image 3A). A guinea worm case containment center was established to assist with management of a disease outbreak. Traditionally, extraction is achieved by wrapping the worm on a small stick or moist bandage and slowly winding (Image 3B). The process is painful and frequently takes weeks. Worms may be 1-m long. *Courtesy: The Carter Center/Louise Gubb.*

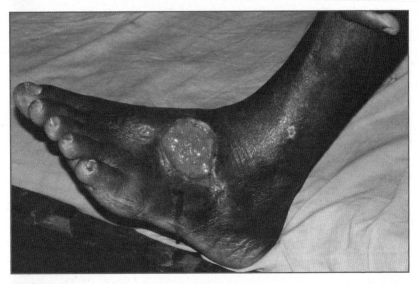

IMAGE 4
Ulceration and secondary bacterial infection constitute alarming complications of dracunculiasis. *Courtesy: Kirsten Johnson.*

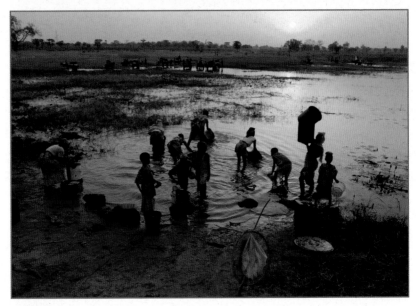

IMAGE 5
Women and children gather and filter water from their community water source. Filtering drinking water is highly effective for reducing guinea worm disease, especially when coupled with other health education strategies. *Courtesy: The Carter Center/Louise Gubb.*

Filariasis, Lymphatic

COMMON NAME

Elephantiasis

BACKGROUND

Lymphatic filariasis is caused by the parasitic nematodes *Wuchereria bancrofti* (accounting for 90% of cases), *Brugia malayi,* or *Brugia timori.* Transmission is via the bite of an infected insect and, after malaria, filariasis is the commonest mosquito-borne infection worldwide. Usual vectors are *Anopheles*, *Culex*, *Mansonia*, and *Aedes*. Humans are the only definitive host. The illness is endemic in more than 80 countries, and the World Health Organization (WHO) estimates that 120 million people are affected. More than a billion people live in parts of the world that put them at high risk. Approximately one-third of infections are in India, one-third in Africa, and the remaining third in other parts of South Asia, the Americas, and the Pacific. Poorly planned urban expansions leading to increased vector breeding sites is responsible for an increasing incidence in many tropical and subtropical regions.

Though death rarely occurs, the severe and chronic physical impairments associated with filariasis make it one of the most important causes of permanent disability worldwide. Marked social stigmatization is a linked complication that further negatively affects children's well-being.

PATHOPHYSIOLOGY

Following inoculation by infective mosquitoes, parasites migrate to the lymphatic system where they mature into threadlike adult worms over a period of 3 to 12 months. Adults measure up to 10 cm and disrupt body fluid balance by anatomically obstructing lymph channels. Secondary bacterial infection likely also plays a central role in disturbing lymph flow. Association of filariae with the endosymbiotic bacteria *Wolbachia* stimulates an endotoxin-like inflammatory response and granulomatous reaction with scarring of lymph vessels. Intramural polyposis and fibrosis of vessel walls ensue and contribute to development of lymphadenopathy and lymphedema.

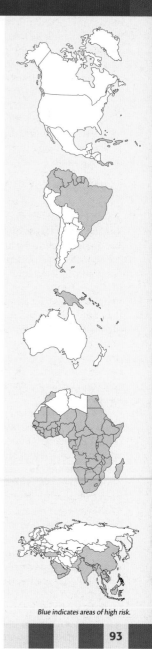

Blue indicates areas of high risk.

93

Life span of adult worms is normally 3 to 8 years and can exceed 2 decades, over which time fertilized females release millions of microfilariae. These tiny parasites surge into the bloodstream at night (exhibiting so-called nocturnal periodicity) and circulate in blood and lymph. If ingested by a biting mosquito, microfilariae have the opportunity to mature into infective larvae and be transmitted to another child during a subsequent feeding. Transmission of filariae by blood transfusion has also been reported.

CLINICAL PRESENTATION

Clinical presentations demonstrate marked variability. Many are asymptomatic. Early stages of illness, as soon as 3 months following acquisition, are characterized by signs of acute lymphatic inflammation including fever, myalgias, headache, lymphangitis, and lymphadenitis. Occasionally, children may only have localized, non-tender inguinal or axillary lymphadenopathy. Tropical pulmonary eosinophilia syndrome is an uncommon acute presentation characterized by cough, fever, eosinophilia, and elevated serum IgE levels.

While initial clinical manifestations usually resolve, successive attacks of retrograde adenolymphangitis (fever with inflammation of lymph nodes and vessels) often occur. Close to one-third of infections result in chronic lymphatic obstruction and lymphedema. The lower extremities are most frequently involved. Genitalia, arms, and breasts are other commonly damaged sites. Consistent with the progressive nature of the disease, older children exhibit higher grades of edema. Pubertal and older males may form hydroceles. Chyluria is possible if swollen lymphatics erode into the urinary tract. Chronic disruption of lymphatic drainage predisposes to ulceration and recurrent superinfections that together result in marked skin thickening and hardening, although these changes take time and are typically not observed in childhood.

DIAGNOSTIC METHODS

Clinical diagnosis can be straightforward. Laboratory confirmation has traditionally been made by microscopic identification of parasites in blood specimens obtained during nocturnal microfilarial migration. This method is still used although the sensitivity is poor, because host immunity is variable and many infected individuals have few or no circulating microfilariae. Adult worms and microfilariae can also be identified in tissue biopsies. In recent years, rapid filarial antigen testing for *W bancrofti* has revolutionized the diagnostic process, increasing sensitivity and allowing for testing at all times of day. Ultrasonography has been used to identify adult worms in inguinal and axillary lymph nodes in children. Magnetic resonance imaging, computed tomography, and lymphoscintigraphy are additional diagnostic tools available in some settings.

TREATMENT AND PREVENTION

Treatment regimens are controversial. Diethylcarbamazine or albendazole in combination with ivermectin is one approach. Diethylcarbamazine and albendazole kill adult worms, and ivermectin kills microfilariae. Early diagnosis and treatment of preclinical infection may abort progression to chronic disease, although this is not proven. Annual mass treatment in communities where filariasis is endemic is effective in decreasing transmission and represents a focal element of the ongoing WHO Global Programme to Eliminate Lymphatic Filariasis.

Once lymphedema is established there is no effective pharmacologic therapy for reversing the underlying pathology. Supportive measures to slow or prevent disease progression include use of compression stockings while ambulant, limb elevation at night or while resting, and frequent limb exercise and massage to facilitate physiological flow of lymph. Close attention to hygiene and regular bathing of affected areas is essential to prevent secondary infections.

Children and young adults with chronic lymphedema are also prone to recurrent attacks of adenolymphangitis. These episodes are painful, limit functionality, exacerbate edema, and promote school absenteeism. Mild cases can be treated with limb elevation and acetaminophen. Topical antibiotics are indicated if superficial bacterial infections develop. More serious infections should be treated with bed rest, limb elevation, and systemic antibiotics.

Aside from mass treatment strategies, prevention efforts should focus on controlling mosquito breeding sites and promoting the use of insecticide-impregnated mosquito nets during sleep.

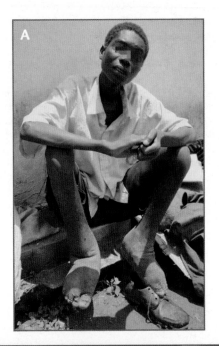

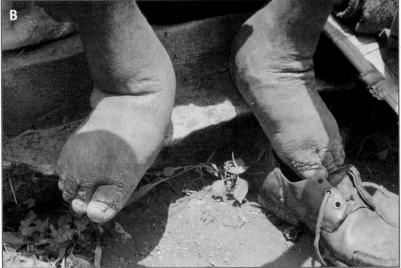

IMAGE 1A, 1B

An adolescent in rural Angola suffers from severe swelling and disfigurement of his lower extremities. He was unable to fit into shoes and instead wore them like slippers around his toes. The disease saddened him considerably. Antiparasitics were administered but unfortunately much of his soft tissue changes were likely irreversible.

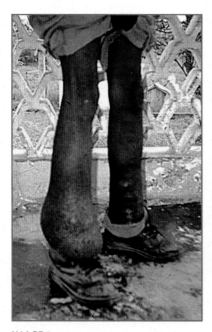

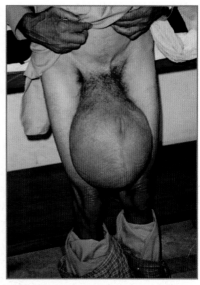

IMAGE 2

Chronic evolution of lymphatic filariasis is often characterized by fibrous thickening and compromise of skin and subcutaneous tissue, which predisposes to bacterial superinfections. *Courtesy: Jose Fierro.*

IMAGE 3

Effects on genitalia are well described. Obliteration of regional lymphatic networks can result in dependent edema and dramatic scrotal enlargement, such as is seen in this gentleman in Nepal. The heavy weight can be completely immobilizing. Surgical intervention is possible but recurrence is frequent. *Courtesy: Kirsten Johnson.*

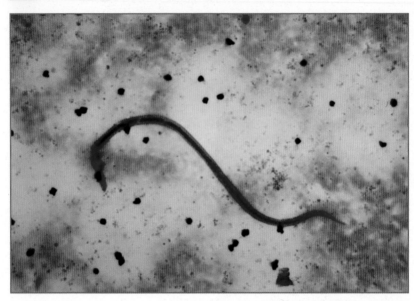

IMAGE 4

Wuchereria bancrofti microfilariae on Giemsa-stained blood film. Each measures approximately 200 μm in length *Courtesy: Centers for Disease Control and Prevention/Mae Melvin.*

Giardiasis

BACKGROUND

Giardiasis, caused by the protozoan *Giardia lamblia,* is the most common intestinal parasitic infection worldwide. Disease is particularly ubiquitous in areas with poor sanitization and unpurified water supplies. In developed countries, the organism is most prevalent in child care facilities, residential institutions, and among individuals with chronic diseases and immunodeficiencies. Humans are the main reservoir of infection, but many animals shed *Giardia* cysts in their feces, thereby contaminating water supplies and contributing to transmission.

PATHOPHYSIOLOGY

Transmission is by the fecal-oral route. *Giardia* cysts are usually ingested in contaminated water. Excystation occurs in the dudodenum, likely in response to contact with gastric and pancreatic secretions and enzymes. Trophozoite forms of the organism attach to duodenal and jejunal epithelium and reproduce by asexual binary fission. Inflammatory changes in the small intestinal mucosa result. Subsequent malabsorption can lead to weight loss or failure to thrive. Some trophozoites encyst and are passed with stool to the environment, where they can survive independently for many weeks.

CLINICAL MANIFESTATIONS

The incubation period ranges 1 to 4 weeks. Children may be asymptomatic, present with an acute diarrheal illness, or suffer a chronic and protracted course of diarrhea. Stools are normally watery and without blood, leukocytes, or mucus, but may be fatty and float when malabsorption is present. Nausea and anorexia are common. Malaise, abdominal pain, flatulence, and dehydration may occur. Fever is rare. Patients with chronic giardiasis can have intermittent bouts of diarrhea interspersed with normal bowel movements or even episodes of constipation.

DIAGNOSIS

Historically, the diagnosis of giardiasis was made by observing trophozoites or cysts on microscopy from

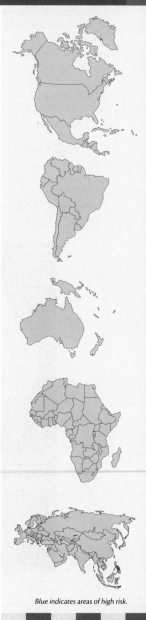

Blue indicates areas of high risk.

stool samples. This technique, however, often requires multiple stool samples and is somewhat labor intensive. Enzyme immunoassay and fluorescent-antibody assays are now available, usually require only a single specimen, and are highly sensitive and specific. Rarely, patients with persistent suggestive features and repeatedly negative stool evaluations may require small bowel biopsy. Abdominal radiography is nonspecific and may show thickening of mucosa.

TREATMENT AND PREVENTION

Management entails specific medical therapy in addition to correction of potential fluid imbalance and electrolyte abnormalities. Empiric treatment is sometimes indicated for children who live in endemic regions with diarrhea and failure to thrive or other signs of malabsorption. Metronidazole, tinidazole, and nitazoxanide all have excellent efficacy. Albendazole and mebendazole, common treatments for helminthic infections, are also effective against *Giardia* and are appropriate alternatives. Treatment failure or reexposure may necessitate repeat therapy. Ensuring good general hygiene is the critical element in preventing giardiasis. Unfortunately, chemical water treatment with chlorination or iodination may not be reliable. Boiling or filtering water is the most effective means for removing cysts.

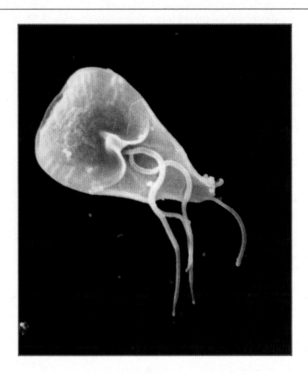

IMAGE 1

The flagellated *Giardia lamblia* trophozoite was discovered in the late 1600s by Antony van Leeuwenhoek, who described the organisms in his own stool specimen to be "animalcules a-moving very prettily." *Courtesy: Centers for Disease Control and Prevention/Janice Carr.*

HIV and AIDS

BACKGROUND

Human immunodeficiency virus (HIV) is the retrovirus that causes acquired immunodeficiency syndrome (AIDS) and, since its emergence in the early 1980s, it has become a major global public health concern. More than 2 million children younger than 15 years were living with HIV worldwide in 2007, and nearly 300,000 died of HIV-related illness. While wealthy countries have demonstrated that the risk of mother-to-child transmission can be dramatically reduced to 2% with advanced medical care, developing world settings have not yet benefited from such progress and collectively account for up to 1,500 new infections daily. Adult disease also impacts considerably on child health, with more than 15 million children having been orphaned by the AIDS crisis. Most children living with HIV are found in sub-Saharan Africa.

PATHOPHYSIOLOGY

Children are infected vertically during pregnancy, birth, or breastfeeding. Less commonly, transmission is by sexual or parenteral exposure. HIV targets cells that exhibit the CD4 marker, including helper T cells and blood or tissue macrophages. Integration of viral DNA into the host cell chromosome is followed either by a period of quiescence, in asymptomatic carriers, or viral replication and subsequent cell lysis. Immunity is critically weakened as the helper T cell population is depleted and pathogens that are normally contained by intact immune defences produce opportunistic disease. Disease progression can be rapid in those infected perinatally. Children and adolescents who are infected at older ages sometimes exhibit a mononucleosis-like acute retroviral syndrome 2 to 6 weeks following infection.

CLINICAL PRESENTATION

The clinical presentation of pediatric AIDS is tremendously diverse. The World Health Organization (WHO) staging system, which grades illness severity between 1 and 4, is a widely used metric for gauging disease progression in infected children. See Box 1.

Nonspecific Manifestations

Children may demonstrate lymphadenopathy, hepatosplenomegaly, weight loss, or psychomotor impairment.

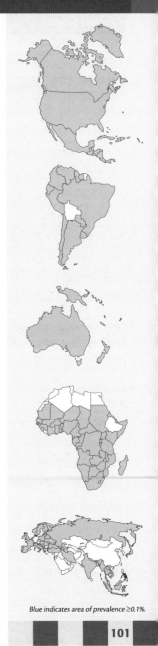

Blue indicates area of prevalence ≥0.1%.

Box 1. WHO Clinical Staging of HIV/AIDS for Children With Confirmed HIV Infection

Clinical Stage 1
Asymptomatic
Persistent generalized lymphadenopathy
Clinical Stage 2
Unexplained persistent hepatosplenomegaly
Papular pruritic eruptions
Extensive wart virus infection
Extensive molluscum contagiosum
Fungal nail infections
Recurrent oral ulcerations
Unexplained persistent parotid enlargement
Lineal gingival erythema
Herpes zoster
Recurrent or chronic upper respiratory tract infections (otitis media, otorrhea, sinusitis, or tonsillitis)
Clinical Stage 3
Unexplained moderate malnutrition not adequately responding to standard therapy[a]
Unexplained persistent diarrhea (≥14 days)
Unexplained persistent fever (>37.5°C intermittent or constant, for >1 month)
Persistent oral candidiasis (after first 6–8 weeks of life)
Oral hairy leukoplakia
Acute necrotizing ulcerative gingivitis or periodontitis
Lymph node tuberculosis
Pulmonary tuberculosis
Severe recurrent bacterial pneumonia
Symptomatic lymphoid interstitial pneumonitis
Chronic HIV-associated lung disease including brochiectasis
Unexplained anemia (<8 g/dL), neutropenia (<0.5 x 109 per liter) and/or chronic thrombocytopenia (<50 x 109 per liter)

Clinical Stage 4[b]
Unexplained severe wasting, stunting, or severe malnutrition not responding to standard therapy
Pneumocystis pneumonia
Recurrent severe bacterial infections (such as empyema, pyomyositis, bone or joint infection, or meningitis but excluding pneumonia)
Chronic herpes simplex infection (orolabial or cutaneous of more than 1 month's duration or visceral at any site)
Extrapulmonary tuberculosis
Kaposi sarcoma
Esophageal candidiasis (or candidiasis of trachea, bronchi, or lungs)
Central nervous system toxoplasmosis (after 1 month of life)
HIV encephalopathy
Cytomegalovirus infection: retinitis or cytomegalovirus infection affecting another organ, with onset at age older than 1 month
Extrapulmonary cryptococcosis (including meningitis)
Disseminated endemic mycosis (extrapulmonary histoplasmosis, coccidioidomycosis)
Chronic cryptosporidiosis
Chronic isosporiasis
Disseminated non-tuberculous mycobacterial infection
Cerebral or B-cell non-Hodgkin lymphoma
Progressive multifocal leukoencephalopathy
Symptomatic HIV-associated nephropathy or HIV-associated cardiomyopathy

[a] Unexplained refers to where the condition is not explained by other causes.
[b] Some additional specific conditions can also be included in regional classifications (such as reactivation of American trypanosomiasis [meningoencephalitis and/or myocarditis] in the WHO Region of the Americas, penicilliosis in Asia, and HIV-associated rectovaginal fistula in Africa).

Common illnesses including otitis media, respiratory tract infection, and diarrheal disease occur frequently in HIV-infected children. Expression of illness often reflects comorbidities typically associated with extreme poverty in endemic regions.

Dermatologic Manifestations

Atopic and seborrheic dermatitis, molluscum contagiosum, common warts, tinea, and scabies are regularly found in all children but tend to be more extensive in those with HIV. Similarly, the course of systemic viral dermatitides such as varicella and measles are usually severe and cause considerable morbidity. Herpes zoster (shingles), verruca plana, and penicilliosis develop almost exclusively in children who are immunosuppressed. Pruritic papular eruption, or *prurigo,* is generally limited to those infected with HIV and occurs frequently in children.

Ophthalmologic and Oral Manifestations

Retinitis from cytomegalovirus or toxoplasmosis can be severe and threaten vision. Chronic unilateral or bilateral parotitis is a relatively common finding. Oral-pharyngeal candidiasis (thrush) should prompt suspicion for immunosuppression when observed in patients older than 2 months. Gingivostomatitis from herpes simplex virus, aphthous ulcers, and chronic ulcerative lesions are possible, and an increased risk of dental caries and angular cheilitis exists. Although rarer, HIV-related oral Kaposi sarcoma may develop.

Pulmonary Manifestations

Pulmonary symptoms constitute a frequent presentation. Pneumonia may be caused by pneumococcus, *Histoplasma* (in Africa, Latin, and South America), *Coccidioides* (in Central and South America), *Penicillum* (in Southeast Asia), *Pneumocystis jiroveci* (formerly *Pneomocystis carinii*), and other organisms. Lymphoid interstitial pneumonitis/pulmonary lymphoid hyperplasia (LIP/PLH) is a chronic inflammatory condition observed almost solely in children with HIV. Onset is insidious and its natural history is characterized by spontaneous remission, periodic acute exacerbations, or progressive hypoxia and respiratory failure. Epstein-Barr virus seems to be a cofactor in LIP/PLH development.

Gastrointestinal Manifestations

Children with HIV regularly experience diarrhea, which may be due to cryptosporidia, microsporidia, isospora, or more common parasitic infections such as *Giardia*. Hyperinfection syndrome with *Strongyloides stercoralis* has been reported. Esophagitis, causing retrosternal pain, dysphagia, and anorexia may occur as a result of candida, cytomegalovirus, or herpes simplex virus infections. Malnutrition is an important feature of advanced HIV and is multifactorial in origin. Nutritional status is impaired by decreased intake related to oral or esophageal disease, malabsorption, increased caloric demands, and poor food access in economically disadvantaged families. Effective nutritional therapy is essential to ensuring optimal growth. Regular weight and height monitoring is recommended, as are annual vitamin A supplements and antihelmintics.

Hematologic and Oncologic Manifestations

Anemia may be infection- or drug-induced (most commonly by zidovudine) and exacerbate preexisting anemia from poor nutrition, iron deficiency, helminthic infection, hemoglobinopathy, or malaria. Thrombocytopenia and neutropenia are also possible. Disseminated *Mycobacterium avium-intracellulare* can present with anemia, neutropenia, fever, weight loss, malaise, anorexia, diarrhea, and lymphadenopathy. In areas where visceral leishmaniasis is endemic, children may have fevers, weight loss, splenomegaly, and pancytopenia. Malignant neoplasms are seen less in children with HIV compared with infected adults, but an increased frequency exists relative to the general pediatric population. Most common are non-Hodgkin's lymphoma, central nervous system (CNS) lymphoma, leiomyosarcoma, and Kaposi sarcoma.

Central Nervous System Manifestations

HIV encephalopathy follows direct toxic effects of virus on neural tissue. It occurs at any age and is most frequently seen in those with rapid disease progression. Infants or young children may exhibit developmental delay or loss of previously achieved milestones. Chronic meningitis typically affects older children with HIV who present with headache, nausea, vomiting, nuchal rigidty, and mental status change; *Mycobacterium tuberculosis* and *Cryptococcus neoformans* are frequent culprits. Focal neurologic findings may stem from space-occupying CNS lesions caused by toxoplasmosis, tuberculosis (TB), or lymphoma.

HIV and Tuberculosis

Children with HIV are at high risk of acquiring TB and developing severe disease, which in turn potentiates HIV viral replication and HIV disease progression. Mortality rates in HIV/TB coinfected children are high. Diagnosis can be difficult because signs and symptoms become increasingly indolent as disease progresses and diagnostic tests (eg, chest x-ray, Mantoux test, sputum smears, and cultures) may be falsely negative. Conscientious clinicians will always consider the possibility of TB coinfection in an HIV-infected child and have a low threshold for investigation and treatment.

DIAGNOSIS

Definitive diagnosis of HIV infection requires confirmation of virus in blood by antibody or virologic testing. While reference laboratories use formal HIV enzyme immunoassays, rapid HIV antibody tests are accurate, inexpensive, and preferable in many community settings. Infants born to HIV-infected mothers inherit maternal antibodies that persist up to 18 months after birth and do not signify HIV infection. Virologic tests by polymerase chain reaction (PCR), detecting HIV DNA and RNA, is necessary for diagnosis in this age group. Infants 6 weeks of age or older who have never breastfed and who have had at least 2 negative HIV PCR tests are presumed to be uninfected.

TREATMENT AND PREVENTION

The availability of life-saving antiretroviral medications has revolutionized the approach to pediatric HIV management, even in the world's poorest countries. The clinical decision-making process for initiating antiretroviral therapy (ART) in infants and children is ideally determined by clinical, immunologic, and virologic criteria. However, it is acknowledged that viral load and immunologic measures of CD4 lymphocytes may not be routinely available in many settings. In these instances, judicious clinical judgment and basic laboratory tests are used.

As a general principle, ART should be initiated in those who demonstrate symptomatic disease and/or immune suppression. This includes most children with WHO stage 3 or 4 disease. Timely treatment is particularly important for infants younger than 12 months, in whom the mortality risk is substantial.

First-line ART regimens normally consist of 2 nucleoside reverse transcriptase inhibitors and a non-nucleoside reverse transcriptase inhibitor. All children older than 4 to 6 weeks at risk of HIV should receive trimethoprim-sulfamethoxazole for prevention of opportunistic infections. Infants exposed to a non-nucleoside reverse transcriptase inhibitor as part of a mother-to-child transmission program (eg, nevirapine) may have developed viral resistance and should receive a regimen based on the likely resistance profile. Updated treatment recommendations for children with HIV in resource-limited settings may be referenced on the WHO Web site (www.who.int/hiv/pub/guidelines/en). Whenever possible, experts in pediatric HIV should be consulted before initiating or altering ART regimens.

The risk of mother-to-child transmission ranges from 25% to 40% without intervention. Antiretroviral therapy for the prevention of mother-to-child transmission, when available, markedly decreases the risk of perinatal transmission during the intrauterine and peripartum periods. Despite the cumulative risk of transmission associated with breastfeeding, exclusive breastfeeding remains the safest feeding option in most regions and should be strongly encouraged unless safe, sustained use of an alternate formula can be ensured.

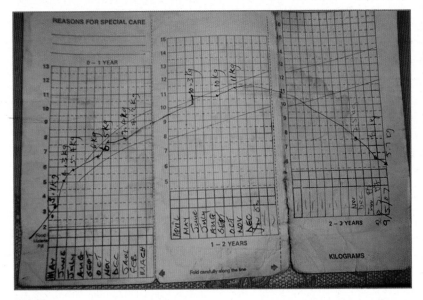

IMAGE 1

The growth curve of child who was perinatally infected with HIV demonstrates a sudden decline in nutritional status at 20 months of age. This unfortunate pattern is common and may result from onset of opportunistic infections, loss of an HIV-infected parent, or sometimes sibling birth and threatened food security. Failure to thrive or sudden weight loss may be the first manifestation of pediatric HIV. *Courtesy: Rebecca Bell and Julie Herlihy.*

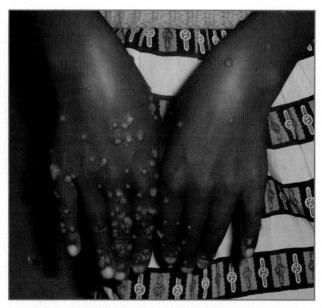

IMAGE 2
Severe common warts, verruca vulgaris, afflict a 13-year-old HIV-infected girl in sub-Saharan Africa. *Courtesy: Elizabeth Dufort.*

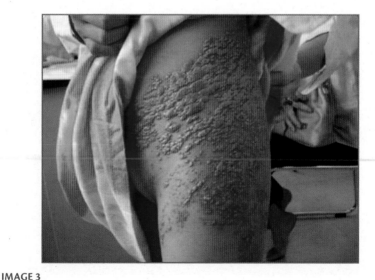

IMAGE 3
Herpes zoster (shingles) in a child with HIV appears as vesicles clustered on an erythematous base in a dermatomal pattern. HIV-infected individuals are at risk of multidermatomal and dissmeninated zoster. *Courtesy: Ung Vibol.*

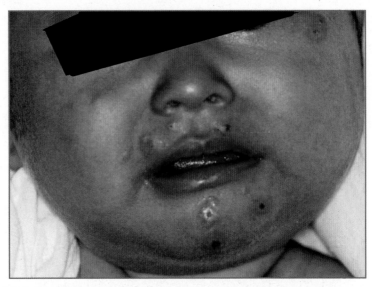

IMAGE 4

An infant in Thailand suffers penicilliosis due to infection with *Penicillium marneffei*. This opportunistic infection develops regularly in HIV-infected children in Southeast Asia. The clinical features include fever, skin lesions, weight loss, anemia, and often lymphadenopathy or hepatosplenomegaly. Papules or nodules are characterized by a necrotic or umbilicated center. *Courtesy: Virat Sirisanthana.*

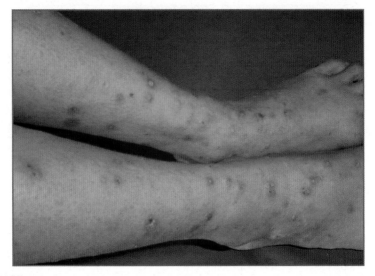

IMAGE 5

Pruritic papular eruptions (prurigo) usually affect the extremities, although lesions can also occur on the trunk. Excoriations are often visible due to associated pruritis. *Courtesy: Ung Vibol.*

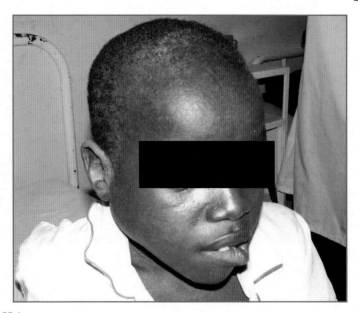

IMAGE 6

An 11-year-old boy in sub-Saharan Africa presents with chronic parotitis due to HIV infection, a condition that occurs with relative frequency in children with HIV. Unilateral or bilateral painless enlargement of the parotid gland is typical. *Courtesy: Elizabeth Dufort.*

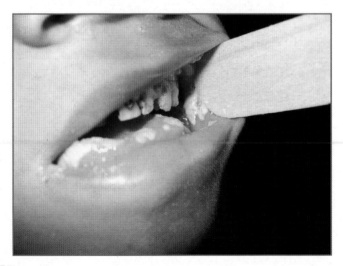

IMAGE 7

Oral thrush (candidiasis) and severe dental caries are noted in a child with HIV in Southeast Asia. *Courtesy: Ung Vibol.*

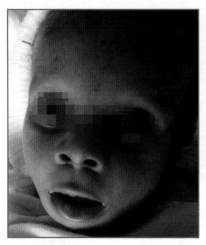

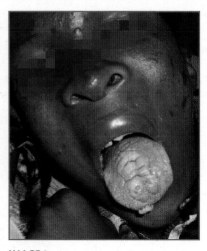

IMAGE 8

Angular cheilitis is common in HIV-infected children and may be caused by fungal or bacterial infection, or zinc deficiency. *Courtesy: Kimball Prentiss.*

IMAGE 9

Kaposi sarcoma of the tongue is possible, although it is not common. *Courtesy: Rebecca Bell.*

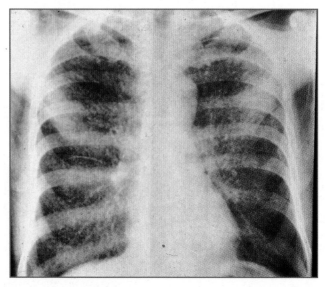

IMAGE 10

Radiographic findings of *Pneumocystis jiroveci* pneumonia include bilateral interstitial infiltrates. Infants are at particularly high risk of developing *P jiroveci* pneumonia regardless of CD4 count. The typical presentation is acute or subacute in onset and frequently includes cough, tachypnea, and significant hypoxia. *Courtesy: Winstone Nyandiko.*

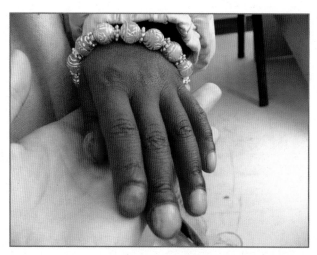

IMAGE 11

Digital clubbing is apparent in an HIV-infected 8-year-old girl in sub-Saharan Africa who has chronic cough, hypoxemia, and a diagnosis of lymphoid interstitial pneumonitis. She had been previously treated 3 times for presumed miliary tuberculosis without clinical or radiographic improvement. *Courtesy: Elizabeth Dufort and Theresa Reich.*

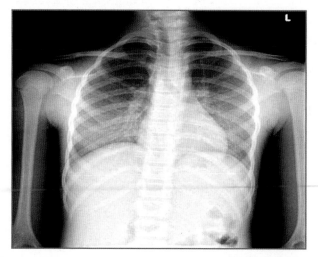

IMAGE 12

A 12-year-old girl in West Africa with congenital HIV is found to have lymphoid interstitial pneumonitis (LIP). Her diagnosis was confirmed by pathologic examination and Epstein-Barr virus polymerase chain reaction positivity of lung biopsy tissue. The radiologic findings of LIP may be easily confused with *Pneumocystis jiroveci* pneumonia or miliary tuberculosis. *P jiroveci* pneumonia is typically more acute in onset. This radiograph displays the symmetrical bilateral reticulonodular interstitial infiltrates seen with LIP. *Courtesy: Elizabeth Dufort.*

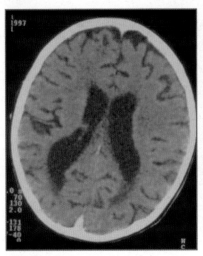

IMAGE 13
Computed tomography of an 8-year-old boy with HIV reveals generalized brain atrophy consistent with HIV encephalopathy. *Courtesy: Ung Vibol.*

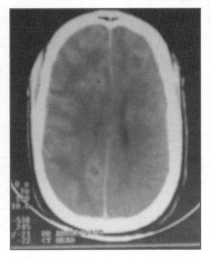

IMAGE 14
Multiple ring-enhancing lesions, typical of central nervous system toxoplasmosis, are seen in this HIV-infected patient with focal neurologic deficits living in sub-Saharan Africa. *Courtesy: Rajesh Vedanthan.*

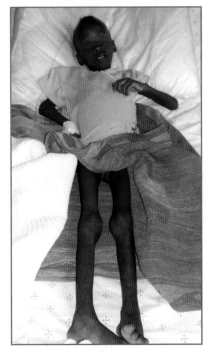

IMAGE 15
The comorbid triad of HIV, tuberculosis, and malnutrition has devastating effects on virtually every organ system. *Courtesy: Keri Cohn.*

Hydatid Disease

COMMON NAME

Echinococcus

BACKGROUND

Hydatid disease is a potentially serious parasitic infection caused by various species of *Echinococcus*. Disease caused by *Echinococcus granulosus* is common in temperate areas of sheep and cattle grazing around South America, the Mediterranean Sea, Africa, Central Europe, Central Asia, China, and Australia. *Echinococcus multilocularis,* less commonly seen in children, occurs in Central Europe, Alaska, the Bering Sea Islands, and Arctic Canada. Disease caused by *Echinococcus vogelii* and *Echinococcus oligarthrus,* endemic in sylvatic areas from South and Central America, rarely affects children. Definitive echinoccus hosts are carnivores, notably dogs, cats, wolves, and foxes.

PATHOPHYSIOLOGY

Definitive hosts infected with *Echinococcus* tapeworms shed eggs in their feces, which in turn are ingested by humans, either directly or in the form of contaminated foodstuffs. Larvae hatch in the intestinal lumen, and penetrate the mucosa to enter the portal venous system. After passive travel to the lung, liver, or other organs, slow development of potentially large cysts occurs.

CLINICAL PRESENTATION

The liver is the most common site for hydatid cyst formation (65% of cases), followed by the lungs. Almost any organ may be affected, and up to one-third of patients have multiple cysts that may involve spleen, brain, and bone. Cysts grow very slowly, approximately 1 cm/year. Small cysts are frequently asymptomatic, and disease is more commonly diagnosed in adults when symptoms develop due to mass effect or rupture. Hepatic cysts are often identified as a result of hepatomegaly or a palpable right upper quadrant mass. Mild nausea or abdominal pain is sometimes present. Colic and jaundice may develop in cases of biliary tract obstruction. Pulmonary cysts are generally symptomatic, with patients experiencing cough, chest pain, and occasionally hemoptysis. Cysts in the central nervous

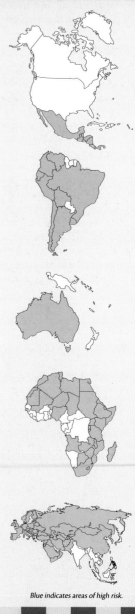

Blue indicates areas of high risk.

system can cause symptoms even when small. Rupture of cysts at any location can lead to severe allergic reactions or anaphylaxis, and any cyst may develop secondary bacterial infection.

DIAGNOSIS

Radiologic studies that demonstrate a cystic lesion in a child with a history of exposure to dogs in an endemic area is highly suggestive of *E granulosis* disease. Pulmonary cysts are readily seen with radiography, whereas abdominal organ cysts are more easily visualized with ultrasound or computed tomography. Cysts are frequently multiloculated and may have flowing echogenic material noted during the ultrasound examination (so-called hydatid sand). Serologic studies are not highly sensitive. Examining fluid obtained via percutaneous aspiration of cysts may reveal tapeworm protoscoleces.

TREATMENT AND PREVENTION

Antihelmintic drugs, particularly albendazole and mebendazole, are effective for treating small (<7 mm), uncomplicated cysts. Larger cysts require more invasive intervention in addition to medical therapy. PAIR, an acronym denoting percutaneous aspiration, infusion of scolicidal agents such as hypertonic saline or 95% ethanol, and re-aspiration, has been advocated but should be avoided when the biliary tract is involved due to the risk of sclerosing cholangitis. PAIR is also contraindicated for pulmonary cysts. Conventional surgery to remove cysts is possible, although care should be taken to avoid spillage of cystic material. The mainstay of prevention is meticulous hygiene, especially around animal hosts and their feces. Periodic deworming of at-risk dogs with praziquantel is also effective.

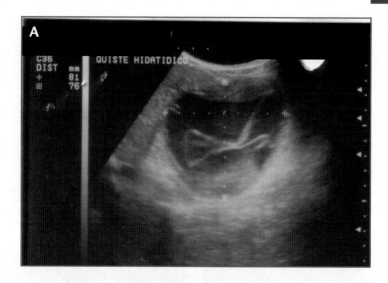

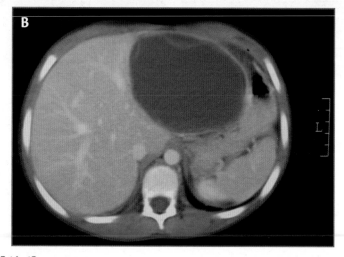

IMAGE 1A, 1B

A 12-year-old girl with a hepatic hydatid cyst identified by a serpent or floating membrane sign on abdominal ultrasound (Image 2A). Detached, floating, inner cyst membranes are also visible on abdominal computerized tomography scan (Image 2B). The entire left liver lobule was occupied by this hydatid cyst. *Courtesy: Javier Santisteban-Ponce.*

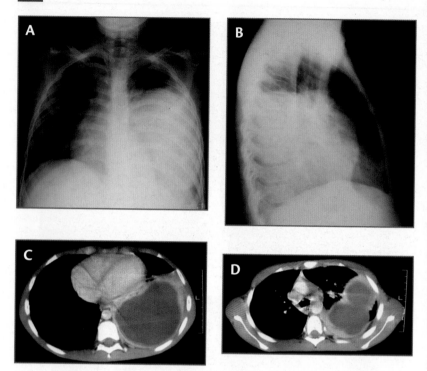

IMAGE 2A–2D

A 12-year-old boy with a left lung hydatid cyst presenting as a large round opacity on chest radiograph (Image 1A and 1B). Computerized axial tomography reveals an ovoid-shaped cyst that is bilobular at the apex (Image 1C and 1D). Mediastinal structures are deviated slightly to the right. *Courtesy: Javier Santisteban-Ponce.*

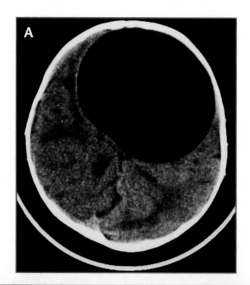

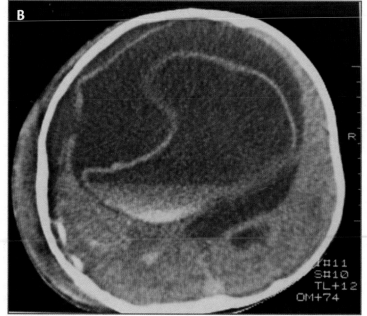

IMAGE 3A, 3B

A girl with a cerebral hydatid cyst (Image 3A). Note the smooth border and fluid density similar to cerebrospinal fluid. She was initially misdiagnosed as having an arachnoid cyst. Cerebral hydatid cysts rarely show ring enhancement nor surrounding edema. Four years later, the same girl experienced a closed traumatic brain injury. The inner membrane of the cyst ruptured and the surrounding tissue bled (Image 3B). *Courtesy: Edgar Morales-Landeo.*

Hypothyroidism, Congenital

COMMON NAME

Cretinism

BACKGROUND

Endemic congenital hypothyroidism is an iodine deficiency disorder that constitutes one of the most important preventable causes of brain damage worldwide. Young infants deficient in thyroid hormone, a critical factor for normal growth and development, endure lasting and devastating mental retardation. Children in neighboring families may also be affected and, in its most extreme form, widespread disease can lead to reduced cognitive capacity of entire communities, causing diminished economic productivity and a self-perpetuating cycle of underachievement. While endemic hypothyroidism is technically easy to prevent, many populations continue to be at high risk, particularly those in selected parts of Asia, Africa, and South America. Congenital hypothyroidism can also occur from genetic and sporadic factors that lead to abnormal development or function of the fetal thyroid gland.

PATHOPHYSIOLOGY

In many parts of the world, iodine is present in soil and found in groundwater and common crops. The thyroid gland uses iodine and tyrosine to produce the thyroid hormones thyroxine (T_4) and triiodothyronine (T_3), which are vital for basal metabolic processes and nervous system development. Conditions associated with reduced sources of natural iodine include overgrazing of livestock, soil erosion from vegetation, and tree loss. When human iodine levels fall, thyroid hormone production is impaired. Goiter, or thyroid gland hypertrophy, results in children and adults with hypothyroidism as the thyroid gland desperately attempts to compensate. The most crucial period for brain development in young children and therefore a particularly dangerous time to be hypothyroid is from the second trimester of pregnancy through the first several years of life.

CLINICAL MANIFESTATIONS

Maternal hypothyroidism during pregnancy may cause spontaneous abortions or stillbirths. Infants born to

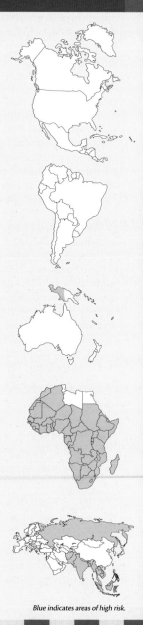

Blue indicates areas of high risk.

hypothyroid mothers are asymptomatic, have evidence of mild disease, or demonstrate severe anomalies. Typical signs include myxedema; mottled, cool, dry skin; coarse facial features; macroglossia; large anterior fontanelle and persistent posterior fontanelle; and umbilical hernia. Excessive sleepiness, feeding difficulties, low muscle tone, constipation, prolonged jaundice, and hypothermia may occur. With time, poor growth and developmental delay are apparent. Mental retardation can be profound. Most untreated individuals will have IQs below 80. Neurologic problems sometimes include spasticity and gait abnormalities. Children may also be dysarthric or mute.

DIAGNOSIS

Assessing thyroid size is useful for determining the presence or extent of iodine deficiency within a particular community. In older children and adults, ultrasound or biochemical markers (such as thyroid-stimulating hormone, thyroglobulin, thyroid hormone, and urinary iodine levels) may be helpful where available. A dried blood spot thyroglobulin assay has also been developed to assist with field identification of iodine deficiency. Diagnosis of affected infants can be made clinically by physical examination in endemic areas.

TREATMENT AND PREVENTION

Ensuring adequate maternal thyroid levels is the best approach for preventing childhood disease. In infants with clinically apparent illness, urgent thyroid hormone replacement and maintenance therapy are indicated to prevent further impairment.

Recommended daily iodine intake is 90 µg for preschool children, 120 µg for schoolchildren, 150 µg for adolescents, and 250 µg for pregnant and lactating women. Universal salt iodization has become the internationally recognized standard for preventing iodine deficiency disorders given its reassuring safety profile, cost-effectiveness, and sustainability. Salt producers and distributors are key partners in this strategy. For those populations with insufficient access to iodized salt, targeted supplementation of vulnerable groups should be strongly considered.

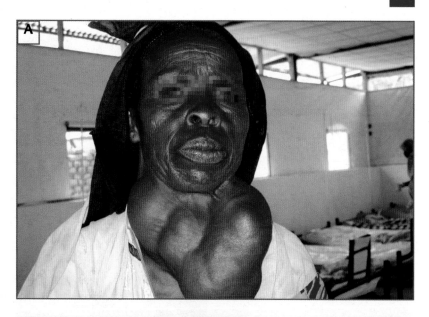

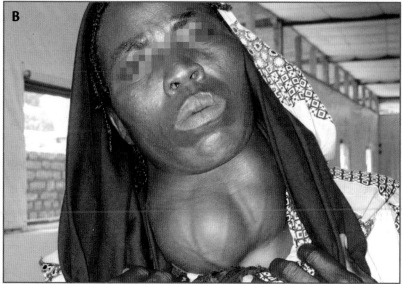

IMAGE 1A, 1B

A mother (Image 1A) and her daughter (Image 1B) in Darfur, Sudan, have endemic hypothyroidism. In all likelihood, their entire village is affected. Many regions that previously suffered from high rates of iodine deficiency disorders have successfully targeted the disease with implementation of salt iodization programs. Countries in conflict, however, have poorly functioning preventive health systems.

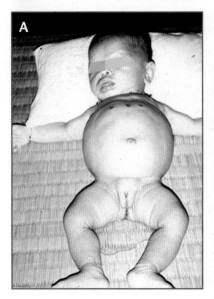 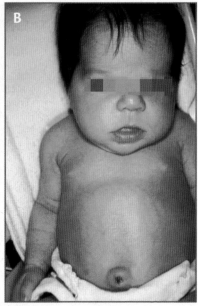

IMAGE 2A, 2B

Macroglossia, coarse facial features, and an umbilical hernia are evident in newborns with congenital hypothyroidism. *Courtesy: Marlene Goodfriend (Image 2A) and Centers for Disease Control and Prevention (Image 2B).*

Leishmaniasis, Cutaneous

COMMON NAMES

Aleppo boil, Baghdad boil, Espundia, Orient boil, Saldana

BACKGROUND

Cutaneous leishmaniasis (CL) is caused by the obligate intracellular protozoa *Leishmania* and is acquired by the bite of a phlebotamine sandfly. Cutaneous leishmaniasis represents a major public health problem worldwide, with 12 million people currently affected and up to 1.5 million new cases developing each year. More than 20 species cause human disease. New World CL is endemic in the Americas from the southern United States (Texas) to Central and South America, and is most commonly caused by *Leishmania mexicana*, *Leishmania mexicana amazonensis*, *Leishmania viannia braziliensis*, *Leishmania vianna peruviana*, *Leishmania vianna guyanensis*, and *Leishmania vianna panamensis*. Old World CL occurs in southern Europe, the Middle East, Asia, and Africa, primarily from *Leishmania major*, *Leishmania tropica*, and *Leishmania aethiopica*. Bolivia, Brazil, Peru, Afghanistan, Iran, Saudi Arabia, and Syria have a particularly high incidence of disease. Rural villagers, agricultural workers, and military personnel are among those at greater risk of infection.

Reemergence of CL in recent years is a consequence of global environmental changes, poorly planned urbanization and population migrations, and altered patterns of host immunity. The vector is a female *Lutzomyia* (New World) or *Phlebotomus* (Old World) sandfly, which typically inhabits wooded areas, rodent burrows, and peridomestic rubbish. They are tiny insects, most active after dark, that rarely travel more than 50 m from their breeding site. Mammals constitute the main disease reservoir—chiefly small rodents but also humans and occasionally dogs.

PATHOPHYSIOLOGY

The *Leishmania* life cycle consists of an infective (promastigote) stage and a host-tissue (amastigote) stage. Sandflies take in amastigotes while feeding from an infected host or reservoir animal. Over a period of 1 to 2 weeks, amastigotes transform into metacyclic

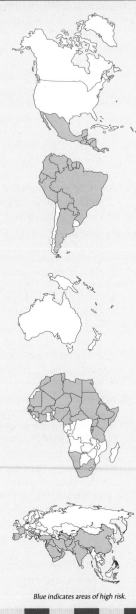

Blue indicates areas of high risk.

promastigotes in the sandfly's intestinal lumen and travel to the insect's proboscis. Promastigotes are inoculated into a new host during the next blood meal. Sandflies are able to transmit the parasite for the remainder of their 2-week life span.

Following inoculation into humans, promastigotes are phagocytosed by cutaneous macrophages. Inside, they convert to amastigotes that multiply rapidly by binary fission. Infected macrophages burst and release high numbers of amastigotes that enter neighboring macrophages, where the cycle is repeated. In CL, the process generally remains localized near the bite site. The ultimate fate of the parasite and the clinical manifestations that develop are thought to be dependent on poorly understood, complex parasite-host interactions. Infection does not provide complete immunity.

CLINICAL PRESENTATION

The classic lesion of CL begins after a 1- to 2-week incubation as an erythematous and painless papule that evolves into a nodule and then a single, large ulceration. Ulcers are 0.5 to 3 cm in diameter, sometimes described as *wet* (with a serous exudate) or *dry* (crusted), and are recognizable by their characteristic central depression and raised, indurated border. Multiple ulcers may occur. Lesions often persist for many months. Slow spontaneous healing results in a flat, atrophic scar.

Diffuse CL is a rare variant resembling lepromatous leprosy, in which multiple cutaneous nodules and plaques develop without ulceration. Leishmaniasis recidivans, found in Iran and Iraq, predominantly affects the face and waxes and wanes over decades.

Mucosal leishmaniasis, or espundia, is a severe complication in 5% to 10% of patients with New World CL. Contiguous, lymphatic, or hematogenous dissemination of amastigotes to the nasal or oropharyngeal mucosa usually occurs after the primary lesion has healed. Chronic nasal congestion may be an early sign. Granulomatous ulcerations result in extensive destruction of facial structures including the nasal septum and palate. Laryngeal involvement is possible.

DIAGNOSIS

Parasitological diagnosis is made by demonstrating amastigotes in Giemsa-stained touch preparations of tissue specimens obtained from the raised border of ulcers. *Leishmania* can also be cultured from these specimens on special media or detected by polymerase chain reaction. Serologic assays exist but anti-leishmanial titers may be low or absent in immunocompromised children and those with uncomplicated CL. Moreover, cross-reactive antibodies may be present in trypanosomiasis, tuberculosis, leprosy, and other conditions. The leishmanin, or Montenegro, skin test is an intradermal injection of promastigote antigen that produces a cutaneous reaction at 48 hours in most patients with established or healed CL and mucosal leishmaniasis. The skin test may be falsely negative in diffuse CL disease.

TREATMENT AND PREVENTION

The goal of treatment in CL is to limit tissue damage and prevent mucosal disease. An association exists between specific *Leishmania* species and treatment outcomes. Small lesions caused by typically non-destructive species generally heal spontaneously and may not require specific treatment. Anti-*Leishmania* therapy is indicated for immunocompromised children and those with multiple, progressive, or dangerously positioned ulcers. First-line management is pentavalent antimony administered intralesionally, intramuscularly, or intravenously for up to 4 weeks. Failure rates for the initial course range from 10% to 40%, and many children require re-treatment. Amphotericin B, pentamidine, paromomycin, and ketoconazole are common second-line agents. Topical imiquimod cream administered every other day may accelerate lesion healing and improve scar quality. Interferon is sometimes recommended for diffuse CL. Mucosal leishmaniasis is treated aggressively with prolonged parenteral pentavalent antimony.

The psychological effects of poor aesthetics are of special concern in children. Prompt recognition and therapy are crucial for limiting the negative cosmetic impact of CL. Vector control programs, management of animal reservoir hosts, and protective practices against insect bites are important preventive strategies. Use of insecticide-treated bednets while sleeping in endemic areas is effective if the net mesh is sufficiently fine (minimum 18 holes to the inch) to impede tiny sandflies.

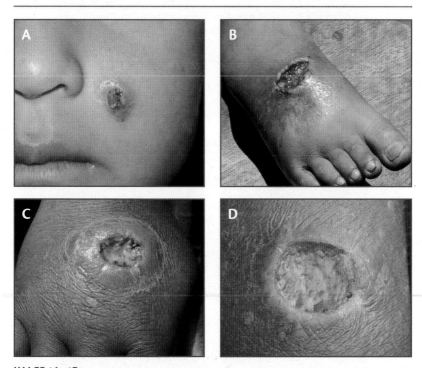

IMAGE 1A–1D
Early nodular lesions in New World cutaneous leishmaniasis (CL) transition to ulceration (Image 1A). A typical lesion exhibits an ulcerated central depression with a raised and indurated border (Image 1B). Wet CL ulcers are covered by serous exudates (Image 1C). Healing during appropriate therapy is recognized by clearance of exudate and progressive defect filling by fibrin tissue (Image 1D). *Courtesy: Alexander von Humboldt Institute of Tropical Medicine Leishmaniasis Research Group, Cayetano Heredia University.*

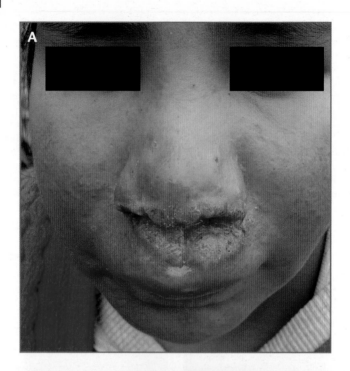

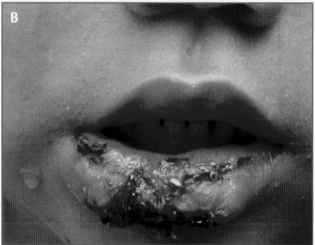

IMAGE 2A, 2B

Untreated New World cutaneous leishmaniasis can lead to mucosal disease, characterized by an intense inflammatory reaction and severe tissue damage. Cosmetic disfigurement can be substantial. *Courtesy: Alexander von Humboldt Institute of Tropical Medicine Leishmaniasis Research Group, Cayetano Heredia University.*

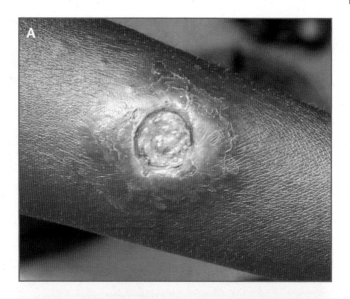

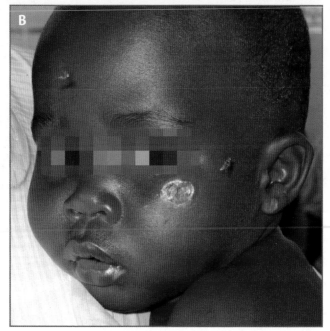

IMAGE 3A, 3B

The odds and rate of spontaneous healing in Old World cutaneous leishmaniasis are dependent on factors such as parasite virulence, host immunity, and occurrence of secondary bacterial infection.

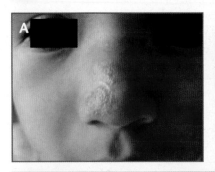
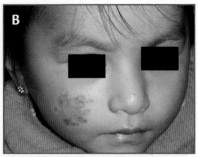
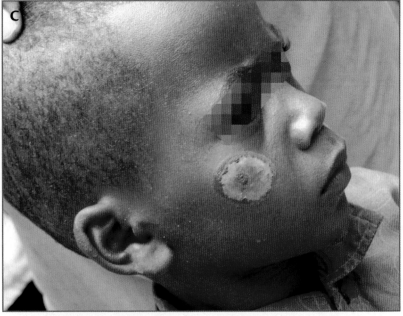

IMAGE 4A–4C
The scars of New World cutaneous leishmaniasis (CL) in 2 Peruvian children (Image 4A, 4B) and of Old World CL in a boy from Sudan (Image 4C). *Courtesy: Javier Santisteban-Ponce and Alexander von Humboldt, Institute of Tropical Medicine Leishmaniasis Research Group, Cayetano Heredia University.*

Leishmaniasis, Visceral

COMMON NAMES

Dum-Dum fever, Kala-azar

BACKGROUND

Visceral leishmaniasis (VL) is a parasitic illness caused by the obligate intracellular protozoa *Leishmania*. Most cases are caused by 1 of 3 species: *Leishmania donovani*, found in South Asia and eastern Africa; *Leishmania infantum*, affecting the Mediterranean and Middle East; and *Leishmania donovani chagasi*, prevalent in Brazil. Rare cases of VL have been associated with *Leishmania major, Leishmania mexicana,* and *Leishmania tropica*. While more than 60 countries suffer from endemic VL, only 5—India, Nepal, Bangladesh, Sudan, and Brazil—account for nearly 90% of the global disease burden. Approximately 500,000 new infections occur annually.

Similar to other forms of leishmaniasis (ie, cutaneous and mucosal), VL is primarily a vector-borne disease spread through the saliva of female phlebotamine sandflies. These tiny insects, of genus *Phlebotomus* (Africa, Asia, Middle East) or *Lutzomyia* (Central and South America), typically feed at dusk. Sustained transmission within a particular area requires large numbers of infected humans or animal reservoirs, usually dogs and rodents. Contaminated needles, blood products, organ transplants, and transplacental exposure are alternative mechanisms of transmission.

PATHOPHYSIOLOGY

Sandflies take up the amastigote form of *Leishmania* during blood meals from infected blood and host the transformation of parasites into metacyclic promastigotes. Following subsequent inoculation into a new host, flagellated promastigotes enter macrophages and multiply. Hosts capable of controlling infection typically do so through a cell-mediated immune response in which helper T-cell activation leads to high levels of interferon-γ production and successful killing of intracellular parasites. Most infected hosts are able to rally this innate defense and keep clinical illness at bay. Patients who develop symptomatic VL seem to have limited cell-mediated immunity and instead go on to

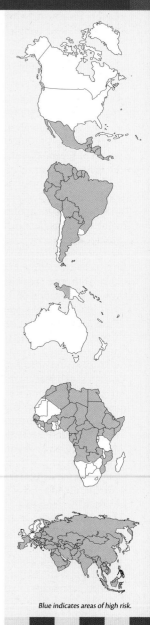

Blue indicates areas of high risk.

exhibit a pronounced humoral immune response characterized by abundant interleukin production and little inflammation. Parasite dissemination through the spleen, liver, lymph nodes, and bone marrow results.

CLINICAL PRESENTATION

Most infections are subclinical or generate no more than mild symptoms. The minority of children who develop the full clinical manifestation of VL usually do so following an incubation period of several months (although the incubation period can range from several weeks to many years). Signs and symptoms are usually gradual in onset and include fever, anorexia, weight loss, night sweats, pallor, wasting, hepatomegaly, and pronounced splenomegaly. Extraordinary abdominal distension may develop. Peripheral edema and adenopathy are possible. In South Asia, hyperpigmentation of the face, abdomen, and hands has given rise to the Hindi name *kala-azar*, or "black fever." Pancytopenia develops as a consequence of bone marrow and spleen infiltration and brings about pallor, epistaxis, and petechiae. Larger hemorrhages are less common. In later stage disease, children develop cachexia, malnutrition, and increased susceptibility to secondary bacterial infections. Many succumb to pneumonia or sepsis. Coinfection with HIV can dramatically alter the clinical course. In these patients, the likelihood of widely invasive VL is increased, the response to therapy is reduced, and the risk of relapse is high.

Post–kala-azar dermal leishmaniasis is a complicating sequela in up to 10% of patients with VL in India and in a smaller percentage of affected African children. Macules and papules first appear 2 to 10 years following primary infection and gradually progress. The face is often involved. Lesions may evolve to nodules reminiscent of those in patients with lepromatous leprosy and can persist for decades.

DIAGNOSIS

Clinical manifestations of VL are frequently difficult to distinguish from other infectious diseases and hematologic malignancies. That said, VL should be strongly suspected in children who live in endemic regions and demonstrate subacute or chronic weight loss, fever, anemia, and splenomegaly. The spleen in patients with VL is often significantly enlarged, soft, and non-tender. Hepatomegaly is normally less pronounced, and the liver is soft and non-nodular. Laboratory testing may reveal thrombocytopenia, leukopenia, and hypergammaglobulinemia.

The gold standard for diagnosis is direct demonstration of the parasite in Giemsa-stained tissue aspirates from spleen, bone marrow, or lymph nodes. Cultures are also highly specific but of varying sensitivity and are slow to yield results.

The Montenegro skin test consists of intradermal injection of leishmanial antigen. A delayed-type hypersensitivity reaction develops in most children who have been exposed to *Leishmania*, although false-negative results can occur in anergic patients with acute VL. Serologic techniques, particularly high-titer direct agglutination tests, are highly sensitive yet less specific due to past exposures to the parasite in endemic areas. The immunochromatographic K39 antigen dipstick is a widely used, easy to perform, rapid serologic test that can be carried out on finger stick or blood serum specimens. Polymerase chain reaction assays exist but as of yet lack commercial availability.

TREATMENT AND PREVENTION

Pentavalent antimony remains the first-line treatment for VL in most parts of the world. Twenty to 40 days of intramuscular or intravenous injections are recommended. Amphotericin B constitutes common second-line management. Other alternatives include paromomycin, pentamidine, miltefosine, aminosidine, and liposomal amphotericin B.

Preventive measures center on avoidance of sandfly bites through repellents, insecticides, and insecticide-treated bednets. It is important that bednets be periodically re-treated to maintain efficacy. Where animal reservoirs play a significant role in transmission, strategies such as deltamethrin-impregnated dog collars have been found to reduce infection rates in humans. Despite advances in our understanding of the parasite and host response, a vaccine for VL remains an elusive goal.

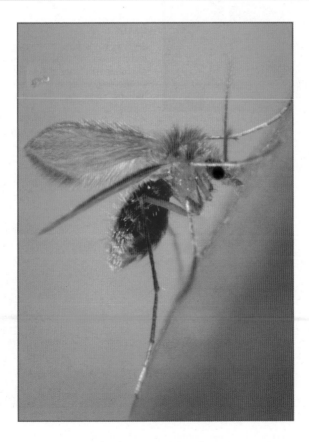

IMAGE 1

A sandfly of the aptly named genus *Phlebotomus*. Pharmacologic substances in sandfly saliva interfere with host hemostasis and local immunity, which enhances the likelihood of successful parasite inoculation. *Courtesy: Centers for Disease Control and Prevention/Frank Collins.*

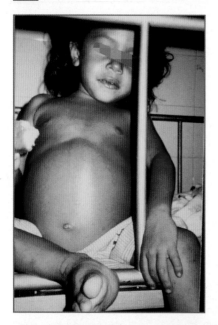

IMAGE 2

A young boy in northern Brazil with visceral leishmaniasis has marked abdominal distention. The "bars" of his bedpost prompt an affecting parallel to his month-long hospital "imprisonment" for daily treatment injections.

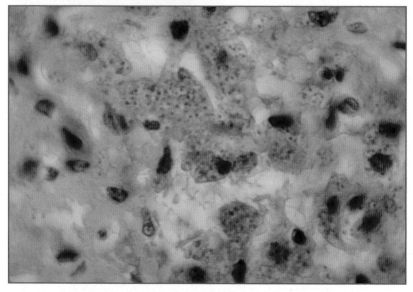

IMAGE 3

Histopathology reveals *Leishmania donovani* organisms within subcutaneous macrophages. Bone marrow biopsy is frequently obtained in resource-permitting settings. Splenic biopsies have greater and more consistent sensitivity, though can be associated with life-threatening hemorrhage. *Courtesy: Centers for Disease Control and Prevention/Martin D. Hicklin.*

Leprosy

COMMON NAME

Hansen disease

BACKGROUND

Leprosy is a chronic granulomatous disease primarily affecting the skin and peripheral nerves caused by *Mycobacterium leprae*, an acid-fast, obligate intracellular bacillus. Patients with leprosy have endured stigmatization and social isolation for centuries, fueled in large part by widely held misconceptions that leprosy was exceedingly contagious and caused loss of body parts. Public health advances and the availability of multidrug therapy have dramatically decreased the prevalence of leprosy in recent years, but some regions continue to suffer from high rates of infection. Seventy-five percent of cases are found in a handful of countries in Africa, Asia, and Latin America. Greatest disease burdens are in Brazil, India, Myanmar, Madagascar, Nepal, Mozambique, and Tanzania. An estimated 2 to 3 million people have been permanently disabled from the disease.

Leprosy disproportionately affects the rural poor, young infants, and the elderly. While HIV does not increase the likelihood of transmission nor prognosis, it has been suggested that accelerated clinical expression of lepromatous skin lesions takes place following initiation of antiretroviral therapy. Aside from humans, the 9-banded armadillo is the only animal in which natural infection occurs.

PATHOPHYSIOLOGY

Mode of transmission remains largely uncertain, although evidence now suggests that spread may be via respiratory droplets. Replication is slow, and the incubation period ranges from 1 to many years. The bacterium preferentially infects macrophages and Schwann cells and favors cooler temperatures, hence its fondness for superficial body compartments. Clinical manifestations are closely linked to an individual's ability to mount an effective cell-mediated immune response to *M leprae*.

CLINICAL PRESENTATION

Leprosy mainly involves the skin, peripheral nerves, and nasal mucosa. Multiple other parts of the body,

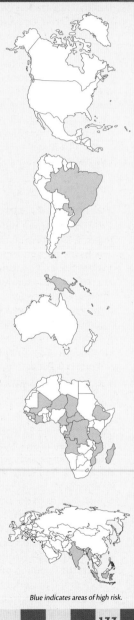

Blue indicates areas of high risk.

including the eyes, respiratory tract, and testes, may also be affected. Several classification schemas exist. The World Health Organization (WHO) has traditionally grouped patients according to number of lesions and skin smear status, a practical approach for settings without access to biopsy technology. Paucibacillary leprosy describes children with few lesions and absence of organisms on a blood smear, whereas multibacillary leprosy refers to those with many lesions and a positive blood smear. The Ridley-Jopling schema takes into account both clinical and microbiological factors and classifies disease as one of the following.

Tuberculoid Leprosy

Cell-mediated immunity to *M leprae* is intact. A single lesion or few cutaneous lesions are present. Erythematous or hypopigmented nonpruritic macules are typical. Peripheral nerves are thickened and tender. Sensory loss puts extremities at risk for unattended trauma, burns, and infections. Scaly plaques with raised borders and central clearing can also manifest. Overall prognosis is good.

Lepromatous Leprosy

Cell-mediated immunity to *M leprae* is markedly reduced. Numerous skin lesions develop. Hypopigmented anesthetic or paraesthetic patches evolve into nodular papules with cutaneous thickening. End-stage findings include symmetrical dermal infiltration on cooler regions of the hands and face, resulting in so-called leonine facies and saddle-nose deformity. Later in the disease, peripheral nerves become cordlike and tender; those frequently involved include the common peroneal (leading to foot drop), posterior tibial (causing toe dorsiflexion and plantar insensitivity), and ulnar and median (resulting in a claw hand deformity). Prognosis is poor in the absence of treatment.

Borderline Leprosy

Demonstrates features of both tuberculoid and lepromatous forms.

Indeterminate Leprosy

An indeterminate form of leprosy falls outside the Ridley-Jopling classification and is characterized by a single hypopigmented or erythematous macule with associated anesthesia. The lesion heals spontaneously or progresses to tuberculoid or lepromatous leprosy. This is a frequent presentation in children.

DIAGNOSIS

Leprosy fundamentally remains a clinical diagnosis with emphasis on a thorough skin, mucosa, motor, and sensory examination. Thorough palpation of peripheral nerves is essential. Any hypoanesthetic skin lesion should raise suspicion for leprosy.

Acid-fast stains of skin-slit smears may be prepared to confirm the diagnosis and to assess bacterial load. The procedure involves scraping the sides of exposed dermis following a local skin incision. Note, however, that this technique is less sensitive in children. *M leprae* has never been successfully cultured, but it is possible to inoculate mouse foot pads for drug resistance testing. Polymerase chain reaction is available at special request through the US National Hansen's Disease Programs.

TREATMENT AND PREVENTION

The WHO recommends chemotherapy with a multidrug regimen of rifampicin and dapsone for patients with paucibacillary leprosy, and rifampicin, dapsone, and clofazimine for patients with multibacillary leprosy. Combination treatment is thought to prevent dapsone resistance, rapidly reduce communicability, decrease the rate of relapse, minimize adverse reactions, and lessen disabilities. Dosage is age-dependent. Recommendations for duration of treatment vary by region. Prior to initiating therapy, potential coinfection with *Mycobacterium tuberculosis* must be assessed because of management implications. Monthly blister packs simplify treatment and are freely distributed courtesy of a partnership between the WHO, The Nippon Foundation, and Novartis.

Patients must be closely monitored during treatment for drug resistance and adverse reactions, including reversal reactions. Type 1 reaction results from delayed hypersensitivity and is associated with additional nerve loss, neuritis, and ulceration. Type 2 reaction, also known as the *erythema nodosum leprosum reaction*, is caused by immune complex deposition and T-cell dysregulation. Multiple erythematous nodules develop in the context of possible fever, neuritis, arthralgias, leukocytosis, iridocyclitis, pretibial periostitis, orchitis, or nephritis. Education of patients regarding these complicating conditions is important, and urgent corticosteroid administration may be required should they occur.

Children must be aware that anesthetized body parts are susceptible to significant injury. Diligent self-care practices are vital. In some regions, reconstructive surgery may be an option for restoring functionality and improving cosmetic appearance.

Leprosy prevention efforts are grounded in (1) national awareness campaigns to reduce stigma and maximize self-reporting and (2) effective surveillance and treatment programs that emphasize early detection and offer multidrug therapy. Close contacts of patients with leprosy should be followed closely. Bacille Calmette-Guérin immunization is likely helpful in conferring immunity to *M leprae*.

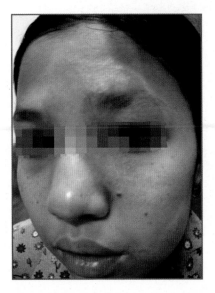

IMAGE 1

An adolescent girl presented with facial violaceous plaques of 4 months' duration. Sensory changes and weakness affected her left eye. *Mycobacterium leprae* was identified in slit skin smears. *Courtesy: Soe Win Oo, DermAtlas.*

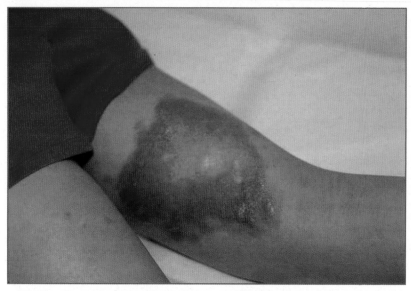

IMAGE 2

A young boy in Vietnam with lepromatous leprosy. Multiple skin lesions and widespread dissemination of mycobacteria occur in this form of the disease. A nodular violaceous macule is shown. *Courtesy: Barbara A. Jantausch.*

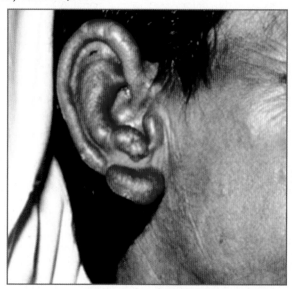

IMAGE 3

Lepromatous leprosy, depicted here in the form of ear disease, is particularly contagious. *Courtesy: Hugh L. Moffet.*

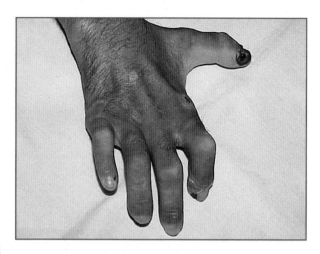

IMAGE 4

A claw hand deformity resulting from thickened nerves in the wrist and hand. Loss of sensation means that wounds, even serious ones, can go unnoticed. Superinfection and ulceration is not uncommon. *Courtesy: DermAtlas.*

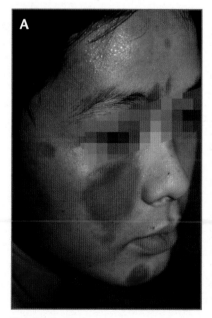
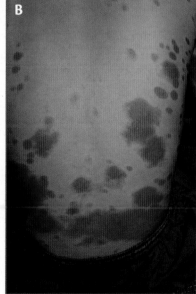

IMAGE 5A, 5B

A Vietnamese adolescent with borderline lepromatous leprosy developed a reversal reaction while undergoing medical treatment with rifampicin, dapsone, and clofazimine. Indurated and erythematous plaques are visible. Prednisone was subsequently administered. *Courtesy: Thanh Nga Tran.*

Loaiasis

COMMON NAMES

African eyeworm

BACKGROUND

Loaiasis is a parasitic filarial infection caused by the nematode *Loa loa*. Disease is most common in equatorial rainforests of Central and West Africa, where prevalence rates vary from nearly 2 % in Nigeria to more than 30 % in parts of East Cameroon. The area of distribution follows that of the *Chrysops* fly, the insect vector and intermediate host. While some African monkeys can become infected with *Loa loa,* the simian strains are distinct from those responsible for human loaiasis. Humans are the only natural reservoir for strains that cause human disease.

PATHOPHYSIOLOGY

The *Loa loa* life cycle is similar to that of other filarial parasites. Inoculation of infective larvae occurs via the bite of the *Chrysops* fly. Over approximately 1 year, larvae mature to adults that reside subcutaneously or migrate to ophthalmic tissue. Adult worms typically measure 3 to 6 cm in length and live for up to 15 years. Females are longer than males. Microfilariae, produced in great numbers by adult worms, exhibit a diurnal periodicity in which their peak blood concentration occurs during daylight hours (when, as it happens, the insect vector feeds). After ingestion by flies, microfilariae travel from the insect's midgut to the thorax musculature and mature into infective larvae over 10 to 12 days. They are then transmitted to a new host during the next blood meal.

CLINICAL PRESENTATION

Most infections are asymptomatic. When disease develops, the most common manifestations are subcutaneous, pruritic masses known as *calabar swellings* that result from locally mediated immune reactions to dying worms or their metabolic by-products. Recurrent tissue swelling can be complicated by the formation of painful cystic enlargements around tendon sheaths. Subcutaneous abscesses may also develop from dead or dying worms. Although it occurs less frequently,

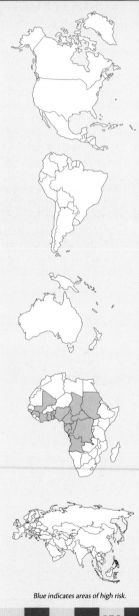

Blue indicates areas of high risk.

migration of adult worms across the eye conjunctivae represents the hallmark of loaiasis. This movement can be sensed by children and may be painful.

DIAGNOSIS

The presence of an adult worm in the conjunctival tissue of the eye is diagnostic for *Loa loa*. Laboratory diagnosis is made by observing hematogenous microfilariae. Thick blood smears stained with Giemsa or hematoxylin-eosin, obtained during the day when peak periodicity occurs, are associated with the highest microfilariae concentrations. Antigen testing kits are now available, and the presence of circulating filarial antigens is also considered to be diagnostic. Serology is less helpful because cross-reactivity exists between different filarial parasites and it cannot distinguish between prior and current infections. Immunofluorescence assays for *Loa loa*–specific antigens and polymerase chain reaction amplification are available but not practical in most resource-limited areas.

TREATMENT AND PREVENTION

Pharmacologic therapy for *Loa loa* usually involves diethylcarbamazine or ivermectin. Allergic reactions can occur from dying microfilariae, and coadministration of corticosteroids or antihistamines may be recommended. Significant neurologic side effects, including encephalopathy, have been reported in individuals receiving treatment for a high microfilarial load. Adult worms in the conjunctivae of the eyes can be removed surgically under local anesthesia. Prevention strategies center on vector control, encouraging behaviors that prevent insect bites, and reducing microfilaremia in human reservoirs.

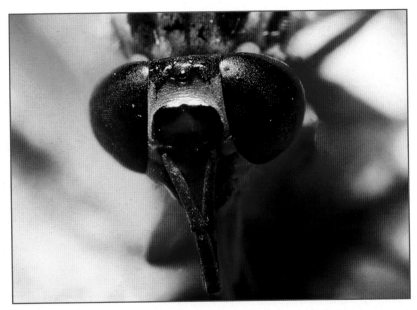

IMAGE 1

Chrysops are a type of horsefly also known as *yellow* or *mango* flies. They lay eggs on leafy plants near water, and their aquatic larvae pupate in nearby mud. *Courtesy: Jorge Almeida.*

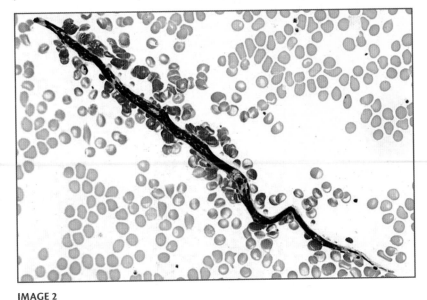

IMAGE 2

Loaiasis was diagnosed by blood smear in a teacher from Cameroon who spent substantial time in forested areas. *Courtesy: Deborah Gold and D. Scott Smith.*

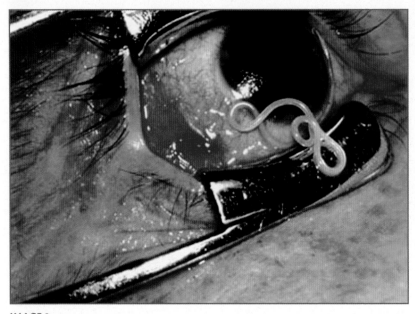

IMAGE 3

A thin, transparent adult *Loa loa* worm migrates beneath the conjunctiva. Intense conjunctivitis, pruritis, and edema may result. Treatment of ocular disease is by surgical worm extraction. *Courtesy: George Waring.*

Malaria

COMMON NAMES

Blackwater fever

BACKGROUND

Malaria is caused by protozoa of the genus *Plasmodium* and is arguably the most important parasitic illness affecting children who live in tropical and subtropical climates. The organism is transmitted chiefly through the bite of female *Anopheles* mosquitoes, although vertical transmission and acquisition through tainted blood transfusions are also possible. Malaria is responsible for 500 million clinical episodes and more than 1 million deaths each year. Africa, Southeast Asia, and Central and South America constitute endemic regions. Overall, the parasite threatens 40% of the world's population in more than 100 countries. Greater than 60% of cases and 80% of deaths occur in sub-Saharan Africa, where the parasite kills 2 children every minute.

Descriptions of clinical features associated with malaria appear in ancient medical texts, including those drafted by Hippocrates near 400 BC. The name itself is derived from the Italian phrase *mala aria* ("bad air"), a reflection of primitive theories of disease transmission. Four species of *Plasmodium* commonly cause human disease. *Plasmodium falciparum* is by far the most dangerous and is implicated in most deaths. *Plasmodium vivax* and *Plasmodium ovale* have the capacity for hepatic dormancy and subsequent relapses, even following seemingly effective treatment. Infection with *Plasmodium malariae* is generally associated with low-level parasitemia and mild disease. A fifth species that infects humans, *Plasmodium knowles,* has recently been identified in Malaysia, Singapore, and the Phillipines.

Parasite reemergence has been inadvertently promoted in recent years by antimalarial drug resistance, civil unrest, unfavorable population migrations, and changing rainfall patterns. Similarly to children, pregnant women are at particularly high risk of infection and complications of disease.

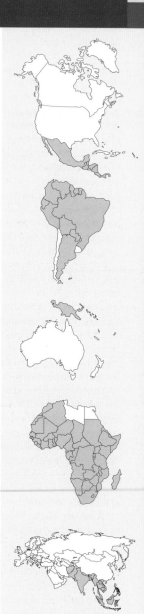

Blue indicates areas of high risk.

PATHOPHYSIOLOGY

Anopheles vectors feed from dusk until dawn, at temperatures from 16°C to 33°C, and below an altitude of 2,000 m. Children are inoculated during mosquito blood meals with sporozoite forms of *Plasmodium* mixed with saliva. Parasites are transported to liver cells in which they multiply by asexual fission and develop into microscopic cysts called *schizonts*. Mature cysts rupture and release thousands of merozoite forms of *Plasmodium* into the bloodstream where they invade red blood cells (RBCs). This prepatent period, the time from mosquito bite until appearance of parasites in the blood, ranges from several weeks (with *P falciparum*) to as long as months or years (with *P vivax* or *P ovale*). Merozoites replicate inside RBCs, ultimately destroy them, and infect other RBCs. As the cycle continues, new crops of fresh merozoites are let loose into the circulation at periodic intervals. Red blood cell lysis triggers release of inflammatory cytokines, resulting in fever and other symptoms. Parasites derive energy exclusively from anaerobic glycolysis, a central factor in the development of hypoglycemia and lactic acidosis that is characteristic of severe disease. *P falciparum* in particular increases cytoadherence of RBCs, obstructing the microcirculation of vital organs such as the brain and kidneys. Thrombocytopenia results mainly from splenic sequestration.

A subset of RBC merozoites fails to replicate and instead differentiates into male and female gametocytes, which are of little pathogenic importance but are crucial to transmission. Gametocytes infect mosquito vectors during subsequent blood meals. The parasite completes the sexual phase of its life cycle in the vector's midgut.

Dormant forms of *P vivax* and *P ovale* are called *hypnozoites*. Children living in endemic regions who survive repeated malarial infections often acquire relative immunity.

CLINICAL PRESENTATION

The incubation period averages 1 to 2 weeks in nonimmune children. Symptoms are nonspecific. Fever, headache, and chills are most common. *Tertian fever* refers to temperature spikes occurring periodically at 3-day intervals that may be seen with *P vivax* and *P ovale*. Less frequent fever spikes, or *quartan fever*, occurring every 4 days, are more typical of *P malariae*. Note, however, only 30% of patients infected with these species present with classic malarial fever paroxysms, and *P falciparum* does not normally induce clinical periodicity at all.

Patients may complain of malaise, fatigue, anorexia, myalgias, and gastrointestinal symptoms. Splenomegaly develops acutely. Hepatomegaly is also possible. Severely affected children can demonstrate prostration, hypotension, hypoglycemia, hemolysis with acute anemia and jaundice, noncardiogenic pulmonary edema, and acute renal failure. Splenic rupture is a late complication usually associated with *P vivax*.

Cerebral malaria is a serious complication defined by (1) coma that persists for at least 1 hour following correction of hypoglycemia or termination of convulsions, (2) *P falciparum* visible on peripheral blood smears, and (3) absence of other likely causes of encephalopathy. Children manifest any combination of decerebrate, decorticate, or opisthotonic posturing; convulsions; abnormalities of tone and reflexes; abnormal pupillary signs; absence of corneal and oculocephalic reflexes; or coma. Hyperreactive malarial splenomegaly, also known as tropical splenomegaly, is associated with a markedly enlarged spleen. The term *blackwater fever* is sometimes applied to patients with extensive hemolysis from *P falciparum,* causing hemoglobinuria and renal failure.

DIAGNOSIS

There is no pathognomonic sign or symptom of malaria. A high index of suspicion is indicated for children with risk factors and unexplained fever or headache. Laboratory diagnosis is based on detection of parasites in the peripheral blood via light microscopy on thick (for screening purposes) and thin (for species identification) blood smears. Immunochromatographic antigen detection tests exist and can be extremely helpful for rapid diagnosis in selected settings. Serologic methods are available but are generally not useful in diagnosing acute disease, and most do not distinguish between distinct *Plasmodia* species. No routine diagnostic test yet exists for *P knowles,* which can only be identified by polymerase chain reaction.

TREATMENT AND PREVENTION

Supportive care of children with malaria calls for rigorous attention toward fever control, hydration, correction of anemia and metabolic derangements, blood pressure monitoring, and seizure management. Specific antimalarial therapy dates back to the 17th century when Peruvian missionaries discovered the effectiveness of Cinchona tree bark. The bark's active ingredient, quinine, is still used today. Most endemic countries have national health policies that outline preferred treatment regimens. Oral antimalarial administration is routine for uncomplicated disease. Parenteral antimalarials are indicated in children who are severely affected. Many recommendations call for combination therapy. Malaria medications include chloroquine, quinine, mefloquine, amodiaquine, sulfadoxine-pyrimethamine (Fansidar), atovaquone-proguanil (Malarone), and artemisinin derivatives. Primaquine is necessary for treatment of infections with *P vivax* and *P ovale* to eradicate dormant parasites.

Pragmatic measures for preventing malaria infection in endemic regions include remaining indoors when mosquito activity is high, wearing covering clothing, liberal use of insect repellent, screening doors and windows, and sleeping under insecticide-treated bednets. Chemoprophylaxis is especially beneficial for travelers who lack acquired immunity. Producing an effective malaria vaccine is a holy grail of global health research. Many groups are working on this critical challenge, and several vaccine candidates exist at various stages of development.

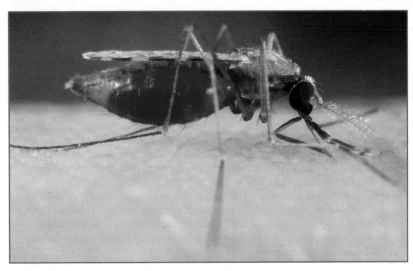

IMAGE 1

An *Anopheles* mosquito feeds. The insect's proboscis is used like a straw, and the successful blood meal is evident in the full, red belly. *Courtesy: Centers for Disease Control and Prevention.*

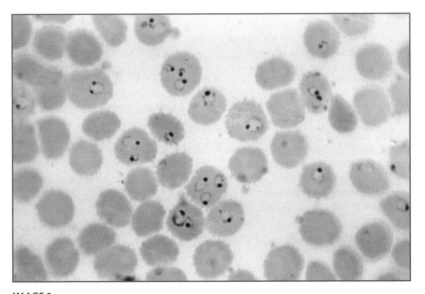

IMAGE 2

Ring-form *Plasmodium falciparum* trophozoites are visible on a Giemsa-stained thin film. The French military physician Alphonse Laveran first described the parasite in 1880 while working in colonial Algeria. Twenty years later in India, Sir Ronald Ross demonstrated the critical role that mosquitoes play in facilitating disease spread. *Courtesy: Centers for Disease Control and Prevention/Steven Glenn, Laboratory & Consultation Division.*

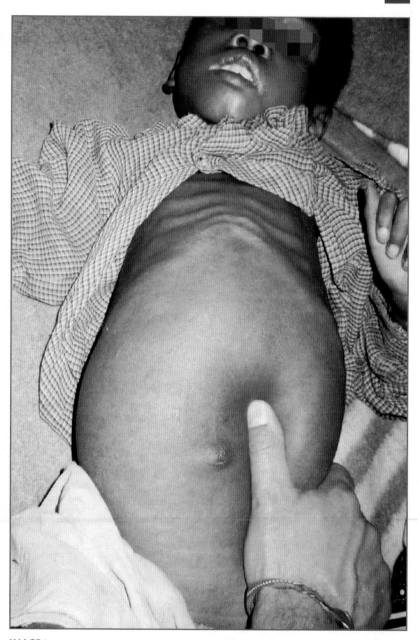

IMAGE 3
Splenomegaly, outlined here by the examiner's hand, is a hallmark of malaria.

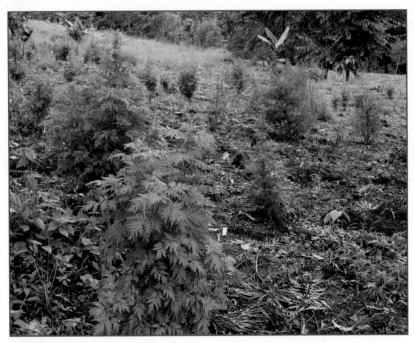

IMAGE 4

A field of artemisia plants, from which highly effective antimalarials are produced. While they are relatively new to "modern" medicine, traditional Chinese remedies have included use of this plant-derived compound for thousands of years. The mechanism of action involves heme-mediated production of free radicals that are selectively toxic to *Plasmodia*. Artemisinin-based combination therapies are generally considered to be the most effective treatment for uncomplicated *Plasmodium falciparum* infections. *Courtesy: Kristian Swearingen.*

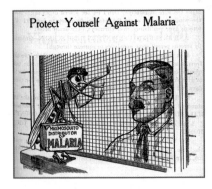

IMAGE 5

Prevention is the best treatment. Bednets considerably reduce the likelihood of contracting malaria. *Courtesy: Virginia Commonwealth University Tompkins-McCaw Library.*

Malnutrition

COMMON NAMES

Kwashiorkor, Marasmus, Protein-energy malnutrition

BACKGROUND

The extraordinary impact of nutrition on global child health cannot be overstated. At least 25% of the world's pediatric population is undernourished, a contributing factor to more than half of the deaths of children younger than 5 years in less developed countries. Children are particularly vulnerable to malnutrition given their high nutritional requirements for growth and reliance on others for food access. Two classic phenotypic presentations exist: *marasmus* (characterized by severe wasting and decreased weight relative to height) and *kwashiorkor* (distinguished by edema).

PATHOPHYSIOLOGY

Malnutrition results when basal metabolic and growth requirements exceed caloric intake. Reductive adaptation attempts to curb further energy expenditure and body nutrient stores are depleted as existing fuel sources are mobilized. Continued tissue starvation negatively influences physiology at every level. Native and acquired immunity are severely weakened. Antioxidant deficiencies allow unchecked free radicals to inflict direct cellular damage. Injury to cell wall sodium-potassium pumps leads to sodium retention and potassium wasting. Hypoglycemia results from exhaustion of muscle glycogen stores and impaired gluconeogenesis. Atrophy and oxidant-induced damage of myocardial tissues bring about cardiac dysfunction. When coupled with fluid shifts from leaky membranes and large sodium loads during recovery, congestive heart failure may occur.

Marasmus is a well-accepted consequence of protein-calorie deficiency, but the specific pathway by which children develop kwashiorkor remains poorly understood. The premise of relative protein deficiency has been largely debunked, and most clinicians now favor a more composite theory involving protein, energy, and micronutrient deficiencies. Exposure to aflatoxins (imposing hepatic damage) and depleted antioxidants (permitting oxidant-induced

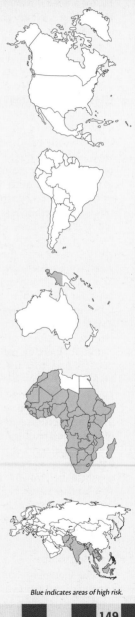

Blue indicates areas of high risk.

149

tissue damage) have been implicated. Decreased glutathione and increased leukotriene synthesis may be responsible for altered inflammatory responses and greater capillary permeability. Together with decreased oncotic pressure from low plasma protein concentrations, vascular fluid leaks may result in characteristic edema and ascites.

CLINICAL PRESENTATION

Marasmus

Children with marasmus are thin and weak. Subcutaneous fat is substantially diminished and wasting is apparent at the shoulders, arms, buttocks, and thighs. Sunken orbits (from decreased retro-orbital fat), skin tenting (from reduced skin turgor), dry mucous membranes (from salivary gland atrophy), and decreased tears (from lacrimal gland atrophy) are common features of malnutrition and should not be mistaken for dehydration. Thirst, thready pulse, history of diarrhea, oliguria, and a sunken fontanelle (in infants) constitute more reliable markers of hydration status. Conjunctiva, palms, and nail beds are pale from anemia. Loss of body fat and decreased activity lead to poor temperature regulation and hypothermia. While localized or systemic infections occur frequently as a result of profound immune function impairment, typical signs of infection (eg, fevers, cough, and pain) may be absent given children's inability to mount vigorous inflammatory reactions. Vitamin A deficiency is associated with malnutrition and manifests with Bitot spots, corneal ulceration, or keratomalacia.

Kwashiorkor

Kwashiorkor is characterized by irritability and apathy in the setting of fluid overload. Bilateral pitting edema begins in the lower extremities and progresses to anasarca. *Flaky-paint dermatosis* refers to dry, cracked areas of cutaneous hyperpigmentation that peel to reveal underlying hypopigmentation and excoriation. Hair is typically sparse, brittle, and reddish in color. Abdomens are protuberant from decreased gastrointestinal motility, bacterial overgrowth and gas production, and weakened abdominal rectus muscles. Hepatomegaly stemming from fatty infiltration may be palpable on examination. Some children exhibit marasmic kwashiorkor, in which elements of both wasting and edema are present.

DIAGNOSTIC METHODS

Dietary intake and social factors represent vital historical data. Weight-for-height ratios are used to diagnose and classify marasmus. Severe, moderate, and mild malnutrition are generally defined by ratios less than 70%, between 70% to 80%, and above 80%, respectively. The mid-upper arm circumference (MUAC) armband is a simple and rapid diagnostic tool that is especially valuable in community programs and for screening large populations. (See sample MUAC and instructions in Appendix C.) Diagnosis of kwashiorkor is made primarily by clinical evaluation (eg, bilateral pedal pitting edema in the context of a consistent history) because edema prevents weight loss and precludes the use of weight-for-height charts and MUAC. (See Appendix B for weight-for-height charts.)

Biochemical testing may reveal hypernatremia, hypokalemia, hypoalbuminemia, hypoglycemia, and hypomagnesemia. If available, blood and urine cultures, cerebrospinal fluid examination, and stool studies may help to identify infected children. Assessment for comorbid malaria, HIV, and tuberculosis is essential. Remember that tuberculin skin tests may be falsely negative due to anergy in malnourished patients.

TREATMENT AND PREVENTION

Addressing the potentially life-threatening complications of malnutrition is an immediate priority. Dehydration, hypoglycemia, hypothermia, infection, severe anemia, and cardiac failure are common at presentation and during early stages of treatment. Some nutritional rehabilitation programs systematically administer oral rehydration solution, antibiotics, Vitamin A, and antiparasitics to all newly admitted children. Folate and iron are replaced after 1 to 2 weeks. Measles immunization is recommended if prior vaccination cannot be confirmed.

Initial dietary management is aimed at preventing further nutritional deterioration, normalizing disturbed metabolic functions, and preparing the body for subsequent catch-up growth. Impaired intestinal and liver function result in poor tolerance of usual quantities of sodium, protein, and fat. Early diets should therefore be relatively higher in carbohydrates. Markers of readiness for advancing nutritional treatment are appetite recovery, resolution of edema, and positive change in affect. Higher caloric loads are then administered to achieve target weight gains of 10 to 15 g/kg/d. Criteria for discharge from nutritional programs vary but should include consistent appetite, weight-for-height ratio greater than 85% to 90%, and an established mechanism for continued nutritional care.

Traditional inpatient therapy of children with malnutrition has given way in recent years to outpatient management. Community-based therapeutic care or community-based management of malnutrition programs treat children with uncomplicated malnutrition through organized weekly or biweekly distribution of ready-to-use therapeutic foods, an approach that has improved cure rates while dramatically increasing coverage and decreasing cost.

Precipitants of malnutrition may differ among populations but are uniformly multifaceted. Socioeconomic and political factors, caregiver education, cultural beliefs, natural disasters, civil conflict, and weather patterns are common factors. Emergent implementation of proven refeeding strategies is a vital imperative while the complex determinants of disease are taken in hand.

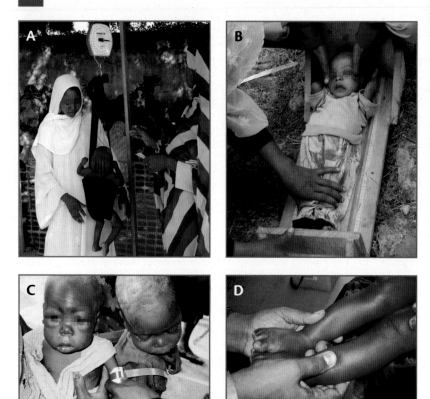

IMAGE 1A–1D

Field diagnosis of malnutrition is accomplished by history, physical examination, and anthropometrics. Weight is decreased relative to height in acute malnutrition, and assessment of weight-to-height ratios using preprinted tables represents the standard method by which to establish the diagnosis of marasmus and determine disease severity. However, while scales and length boards are by some measures easy to operate and maintain, they can still be too complicated and time-consuming for sustained and accurate use in remote settings (Image 1A, 1B). MUAC (mid-upper arm circumference) armbands represent an even simpler screening and diagnostic tool (Image 1C). In children aged 1 to 5 years, the circumference at the midpoint of the upper arm remains relatively stable as "baby fat" is replaced by lean muscle mass. MUAC less than 110 mm has been shown to be associated with severe malnutrition and that between 110 to 125 mm is indicative of moderate and mild malnutrition. Kwashiorkor is diagnosed by different means—specifically, presence of edema (Image 1D). Of note, stunting occurs with chronic malnutrition and is characterized by decreased height-for-age.

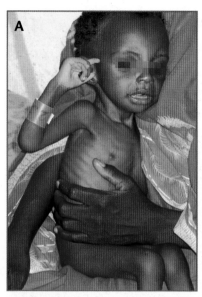 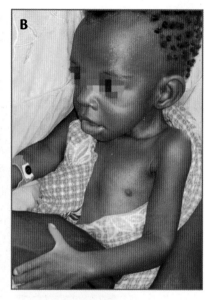

IMAGE 2A, 2B

Marasmus in a young child whose family had been displaced as a result of civil conflict in Angola (Image 2A). Substantial improvement was observed following only 2 weeks of treatment at an inpatient therapeutic feeding center (Image 2B). Tissue surrounding the orbits and rib cage appeared much healthier, and the child demonstrated increased alertness and interactivity.

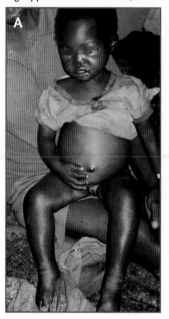 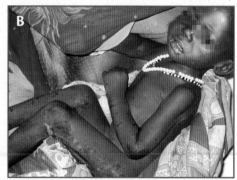

IMAGE 3A, 3B

The term *kwashiorkor* is derived from the west African *Ga* vernacular for a child "who is physically displaced." It refers to children who have been weaned from the breast to accommodate a younger sibling. Kwashiorkor tends to occur in children aged 1 to 4 years and was first described by Cecily Williams in present-day Ghana as a nutritional disease associated with a maize diet. Defining clinical features are edema (Image 3A) and flaky-paint dermatosis (Image 3B).

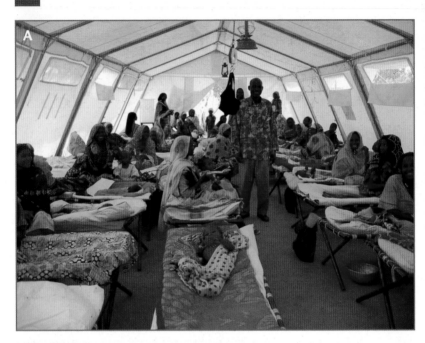

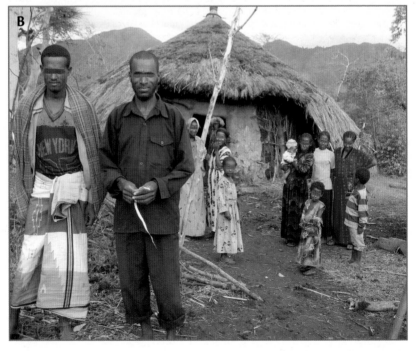

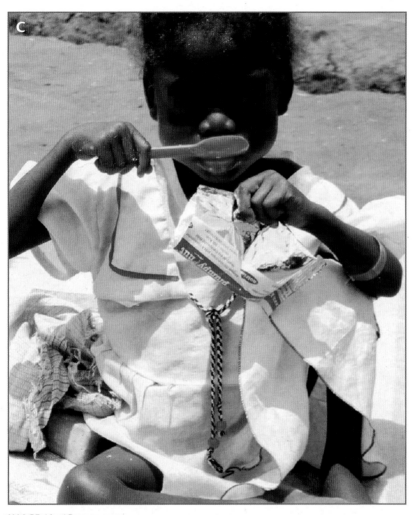

IMAGE 4A–4C

Inpatient nutritional rehabilitation centers have the advantage of ensuring close patient monitoring but are costly and severely limit coverage. In addition, close quartering of sick children can promote nosocomial illness (Image 4A). New trends in management reserve inpatient therapy for malnourished children with complicated disease and treat most malnourished children at home in their own communities. Village health workers are trained to use MUAC (mid-upper arm circumference) and to refer children with suspected malnutrition to outpatient programs that are no more than half a day's walk (Image 4B). This approach maximizes early identification of affected children, who are then provided with a 1- to 2-week supply of ready-to-use therapeutic food and evaluated at regular visits for weight gain. Ready-to-use therapeutic food is a caloric-rich, oil-based paste that can last up to 12 months without refrigeration (Image 4C). Plumpy-nut is a frequently used product produced in France, but local production methods are becoming more popular for obvious reasons.

Measles

COMMON NAME

Rubeola

BACKGROUND

The World Health Organization (WHO) estimates that nearly a quarter million measles-related deaths occurred in 2006, most involving children, making it one of the leading causes of child mortality worldwide. Less developed countries represent the highest-risk settings, particularly within areas of crowding and low immunization coverage.

Humans are the only known reservoir. Transmission occurs by either (1) direct inoculation via contact with infectious droplets or (2) aerosolized spread of virus particles such as occurs during coughing or sneezing. Measles is extraordinarily contagious: virtually 100% of susceptible children develop disease following exposure. Infectiousness is greatest in the days before the onset of symptoms, which compounds measles' ability to spread rapidly.

PATHOPHYSIOLOGY

Measles is an RNA paramyxovirus. After infection, the virus replicates in respiratory epithelium, circulates to local lymphatic tissue, and disseminates hematogenously to multiple organ systems.

CLINICAL PRESENTATION

The incubation period is 10 days. Symptoms begin with an acute prodrome of high fever and malaise, cough, coryza, and conjunctivitis. Severe viral pneumonia may develop. Koplik spots are a pathognomonic enanthem involving the buccal mucosa that appear near the second day of illness and are characterized by bluish-white papules on an erythematous base. The rash of measles manifests on the fourth day, first behind the ears and on the forehead and then extending inferiorly to the face and trunk. Lesions are initially discrete, erythematous, maculopapular, and "sandpapery." Over time, spots often coalesce, fade to light brown, and ultimately desquamate.

While measles itself is self-limiting, secondary complications contribute considerably to its

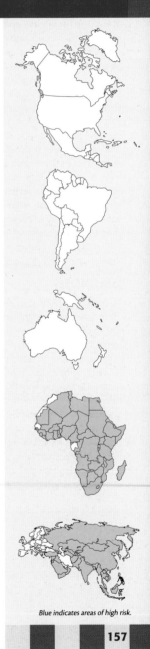

Blue indicates areas of high risk.

morbidity and mortality. Lower respiratory tract infections, severe tracheobronchitis (presenting as croup), and otitis media are possible. Diarrhea may develop early and persist, putting already compromised children at additional risk for dehydration and malnutrition. Measles can precipitate a dramatic plummet of Vitamin A levels and quickly trigger irreversible ophthalmologic events including blindness. Neurologic manifestations usually take the form of febrile seizures, but both encephalitis and post-infectious encephalopathy can also occur. Subacute sclerosing panencephalitis is a rare, late sequela associated with chronic viral contamination of the central nervous system; progressive behavioral changes and cognitive deterioration are hallmarks.

DIAGNOSIS

Measles is a clinical diagnosis suggested by characteristic signs and symptoms, specifically cough, coryza, conjunctivitis, and a morbilliform exanthem. Koplik spots, which are present in up to 80% of cases, assist greatly in diagnosis but are short-lived and may disappear before children are examined. Laboratory confirmation is by serology, demonstrating an elevated measles IgM titer. Testing for acute and convalescent IgG antibodies can also be performed, as can direct isolation of virus from blood, urine, or nasopharyngeal secretions.

TREATMENT AND PREVENTION

Treatment is largely supportive, with special attention to fluid management, antipyretics, and optimization of nutrition. Vitamin A supplementation is critical and has been found to reduce ophthalmologic complications as well as mortality. Antibiotics are indicated for secondary bacterial infections. Overall case-fatality rates average 5%.

Immune globulin prevents or lessens severity of disease when administered to susceptible children within 6 days of exposure and is especially important for infants and those who are immunocompromised.

A 2-dose regimen of oral measles vaccine is highly efficacious, safe, and extremely cost-effective. Unfortunately, the formulation is susceptible to inactivation by warming, and maintenance of an unfailing cold-chain from the site of production to dispensation remains a major challenge of effective distribution. Recommendations for timing of the first immunization dose vary. UNICEF advocates routine administration of the first dose at 9 months of age or shortly thereafter. The first dose may be given to children as young as 6 months in complex emergency situations where risk of outbreak is high. Countries that enjoy low disease prevalence, in contrast, often delay the first dose until 12 to 15 months of age to ensure that development of active immunity is not precluded by persistent maternal antibodies.

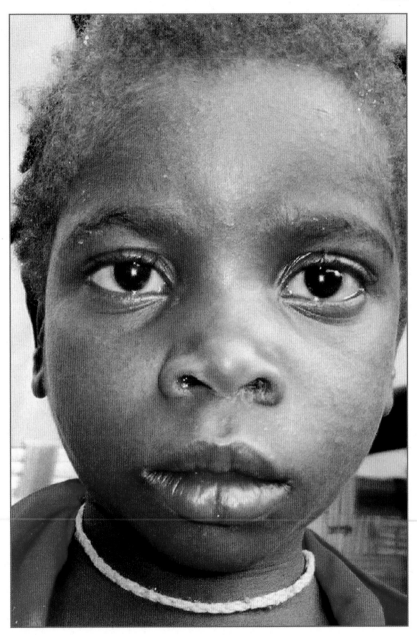

IMAGE 1
Measles rash in dark-skinned children can be subtle. Conjunctivitis and coryza are more striking.

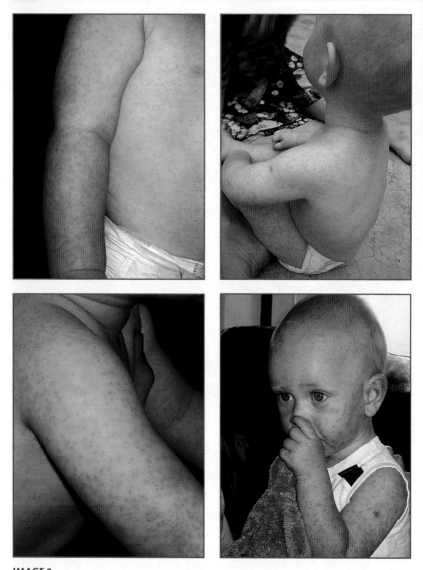

IMAGE 2

The morbilliform exanthem in lighter-skinned children is difficult to miss. This boy acquired measles while traveling in South Africa before he was immunized.

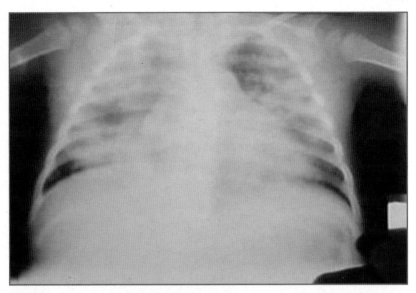

IMAGE 3

Viral pneumonia caused by measles is also known as *large cell pneumonia*, reflecting the histopathologic changes that occur in reticuloendothelial tissue and respiratory epithelium. *Staphylococcus* pneumonia, pictured in this radiograph, is a feared superinfection. *Courtesy: Tina Slusher.*

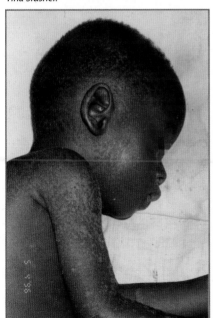

IMAGE 4

Fever in measles is high and occurs early. By the time skin lesions appear on day 4 or so, children begin to defervesce. After several days, measles rash fades from red to light brown and then desquamates, as seen here. *Courtesy: Tina Slusher.*

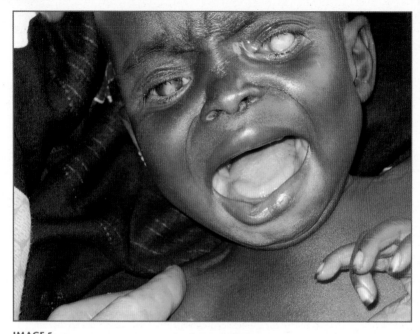

IMAGE 5

Vitamin A deficiency in measles is of vital concern. A cascade of unfortunate ophthalmologic events including xerophthalmia (excessive dryness), corneal ulceration, keratomalacia, and corneal scarring can rapidly lead to irreversible blindness.

Melioidosis

BACKGROUND

Melioidosis is a potentially fatal bacterial infection caused by the saprophytic gram-negative bacillus *Burkholderia pseudomallei* (formerly *Pseudomonas*). Disease is most common in Southeast Asia, is also endemic in Northern Australia, and has been reported sporadically in tropical settings worldwide. Outbreaks were recognized, especially among children, following the Asian tsunami in December 2004. The greatest risk factor is frequent contact with wet soil. Not surprisingly, incidence is seasonal and weighted toward rainy months. Most cases occur in Thailand, where up to 50% of rice paddies harbor the bacterium, and much of the rural population seroconverts by age 4. While children are certainly affected, melioidosis predominantly targets adults older than 40 years, especially those already compromised by underlying illness such as diabetes. A particular association with HIV has not been demonstrated.

PATHOPHYSIOLOGY

B pseudomallei is a resilient organism that can live for years in harsh environments. Transmission is by inhalation or direct soft tissue inoculation. High rates of bacteremia can rapidly develop following infection and are associated with severe inflammatory responses to antigenic stimuli including lipopolysaccharide. The polysaccharide capsule of *B pseudomallei* is another important virulence determinant that contributes to formation of a biofilm conferring antibiotic resistance. Most patients present shortly after exposure, but latency (for months to years) with reactivation is well described.

CLINICAL PRESENTATION

Most infections are asymptomatic. When they occur, clinical manifestations are notoriously protean. Disease may be local or systemic, acute or chronic, and immediate or delayed. In children, suppurative parotitis accounts for approximately a third of cases in Southeast Asia (this presentation is rare in Australia). Symptoms are fever, pain, and localized parotid gland swelling. Ten percent are bilateral. Unlike most adult melioidosis, children with parotitis frequently have no underlying predisposing conditions and respond well to treatment.

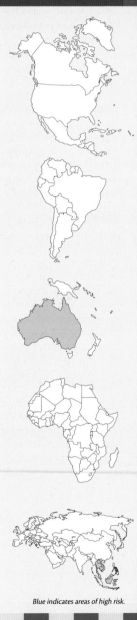

Blue indicates areas of high risk.

Other presentations in children include single or multiple cutaneous abscesses and suppurative infection of bones, joints, lymph nodes, liver, or spleen. Fever is common. Sepsis also occurs, sometimes complicated by pneumonia and, in fulminant cases, death. Focal infections of the central nervous system are possible.

In older populations, airborne spread or systemic pathogen dissemination results in frequent lung involvement. Patients present with cough and fever stemming from pulmonary abscesses, pneumonia, or empyema. Diffuse nodular infiltrates can develop, coalesce, cavitate, and lead to metastatic lesions.

DIAGNOSIS

Melioidosis cannot reliably be clinically distinguished from other bacterial infections, but sepsis and abscess formation in a patient with risk factors should arouse suspicion and prompt consideration of empiric therapy pending microbiological confirmation. Diagnosis is by culture of organisms in blood, sputum, or pus from an affected site. Throat cultures are sensitive and can increase diagnostic yield. Ashdown selective medium is often used, although the organism grows on most agar. It is important to be aware of laboratories in non-endemic settings that may incorrectly identify *B pseudomallei* as *Pseudomonas* species. Due to high rates of seropositivity in endemic areas, antibody tests are not useful in diagnosing acute disease.

TREATMENT AND PREVENTION

Diligent supportive care with attention to fluid management is essential for patients with sepsis syndromes. Abscesses should be drained when possible. Ceftazidime, imipenem, or meropenem for a minimum of 10 days is standard for initial treatment of invasive disease. Defervescence may take a week or longer, even with appropriate antibiotic management, and new suppurative lesions can develop during early treatment. A prolonged oral antibiotic regimen is mandatory following parenteral therapy to completely eradicate the organism and reduce the risk of relapse. Specific recommendations for oral antibiotic selection and duration vary by region; some advocate trimethoprim-sulfamethoxazole plus doxycycline for 8 weeks (in the case of uncomplicated parotitis) to 5 months (for severe or systemic disease).

The prognosis of melioidosis is much better for children than for adults, and rates of relapse are lower. No vaccine is available. Prevention is difficult because contact with water and soil is usually essential to families who live in many endemic regions where livelihoods are agriculture-based.

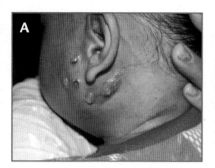 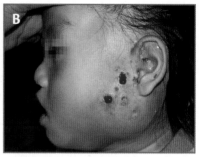

IMAGE 1A, 1B

Unilateral suppurative parotitis is apparent in a young Laotian girl with melioidosis. Areas of spontaneous drainage are visible. *Courtesy: Rattanaphone Phetsouvanh.*

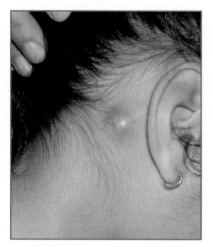

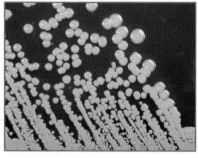

IMAGE 3

Burkholderia pseudomallei in culture. Concerns exist that *B pseudomallei* could be used as an agent of biological warfare given its ability to be transmitted via inhalation. *Courtesy: Centers for Disease Control and Prevention/Larry Stauffer, Oregon State Public Health Laboratory.*

IMAGE 2

While parotitis is a common presentation, any abscess formation in children who live in endemic regions should raise suspicion for melioidosis. Here, disease manifested as a unilateral suppurative postauricular lymph node. *Courtesy: Rattanaphone Phetsouvanh.*

Meningococcemia

BACKGROUND

Meningococcemia is a potentially life-threatening systemic infection caused by the gram-negative diplococcus *Neisseria meningitidis*. The disease is found worldwide, but has a markedly increased prevalence in the meningitis belt found across a wide swath of sub-Saharan Africa, from Ethiopia in the east to Gambia and Senegal in the west. Five main serotypes exist: A, B, C, W-135, and Y. Different serotypes account for disease variation within target populations and between locales.

PATHOPHYSIOLOGY

The organism is transmitted via small droplets. The portal of entry is the respiratory system and the incubation period is short, usually less than 4 days. Multiple *Neisseria* species, including meningococcus, can asymptomatically colonize the nasopharynx. In a small subset of patients, the organism invades the bloodstream and triggers a catastrophic cascade characterized by endotoxin release; microvasculitis; and progression to disseminated intravascular coagulation, septic shock, and death. The complement system seems particularly important in protecting against meningococcal disease, and those with complement deficiency are at higher risk.

CLINICAL PRESENTATION

Many of those exposed to meningococcus will be colonized but remain asymptomatic. If symptoms develop, the most common manifestations are those of meningococcemia or meningitis. Meningococcemia may initially present as a viral-like syndrome, but then progress to high fever with headache, hypotension and, ultimately, shock. More than two-thirds of patients have the classic skin finding of petechiae coalescing into irregularly shaped purpura, frequently with a grayish center. These lesions may progress to purpura fulminans, which resembles a burn and often requires skin grafting. Arthralgias are common. Meningitis can occur either alone or in association with meningococcemia. It presents as do other causes of bacterial meningitis with fever, headache, and nuchal

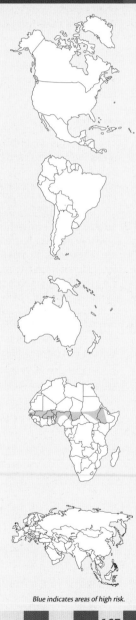

Blue indicates areas of high risk.

rigidity. Mortality from meningococcemia approaches 15% and is lower in cases of meningitis, likely because the child survived long enough to develop the central nervous system infection. Uncommon complications of meningococcemia include adrenal hemorrhage, pericarditis, and debilitating arthritis, which often develops as the patient is recovering.

DIAGNOSIS

The diagnosis is confirmed when *N meningitidis* grows in culture from a normally sterile body fluid, usually blood or cerebrospinal fluid. Isolation of meningococcus from the nasopharynx does not indicate systemic disease. Leukocytosis, leukopenia, or thrombocytopenia may be indicative but are nonspecific. Spinal fluid should be obtained from any patient with suspected meningococcal disease. Cerebrospinal fluid pleocytosis of 1,000 cells or more (mostly polynuclear leukocytes) is typical. In resource-constrained areas, suggestive skin findings in a critically ill patient should prompt immediate empiric therapy.

TREATMENT AND PREVENTION

Parenteral antibiotics are indicated in those with confirmed or strongly suspected meningococcemia. Penicillins remain the standard, but third-generation cephalosporins (eg, ceftriaxone) are also effective and frequently used. In addition, aggressive supportive care is often necessary, including possible fluid resuscitation, vasopressor administration, and ventilatory support. As noted, it is not uncommon for patients with fulminant cutaneous disease to require skin grafting or even amputation of affected limbs. Close contacts of index cases should be prophylaxed with rifampin or ceftriaxone for children, or ciprofloxacin for adults. Vaccines are now available against serotypes A, C, Y, and W-135 and can be administered to close contacts during an outbreak in addition to chemoprophylaxis. No vaccine exists against serotype B, the most common cause of disease in infants. In the United States, it is recommended that all 11- to 12-year-olds be vaccinated with the tetravalent meningococcal conjugate vaccine.

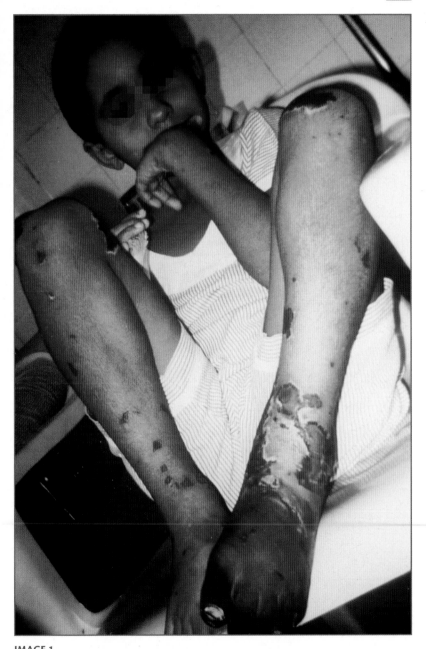

IMAGE 1
Petechial rash in meningococcemia gives way to large pupuric lesions in severe cases. Cutaneous effects in survivors can be permanent.

Molluscum Contagiosum

BACKGROUND

Molluscum contagiosum is a benign cutaneous viral infection caused by the aptly named *Molluscipoxvirus*. Distribution is global but most prevalent in warm climates and crowded living conditions. Transmission occurs by direct contact with affected individuals or via fomites. Lesions are known to spread on the same individual by autoinoculation, hence a minor predilection for flexural parts of the body. Humans are the only known reservoir.

Immunocompromised children are at higher risk of contracting molluscum and are also more likely to suffer from local inflammatory reactions and bacterial superinfections. Fortunately, systemic dissemination does not occur.

PATHOPHYSIOLOGY

This DNA poxvirus targets epidermal keratinocytes, replicates within cytoplasm, and invokes cellular acanthosis (hyperproliferation). Lesions remain confined to the epithelium.

CLINICAL PRESENTATION

Incubation varies from weeks to months, after which appear discrete and firm dome-shaped papules with central umbilication. Lesions typically measure 3 to 5 mm, have a flesh or pearly-white tint, and may be found in clusters. The face, trunk, and extremities are commonly affected.

DIAGNOSIS

Recognition of characteristic lesions facilitates clinical diagnosis. Although rarely necessary, microscopic examination of stained skin scrapings reveals pathognomonic intracytoplasmic viral inclusions (so-called molluscum bodies).

TREATMENT AND PREVENTION

Lesions generally involute spontaneously without scarring after several months, and specific treatment often is not required. In persistent or severe cases,

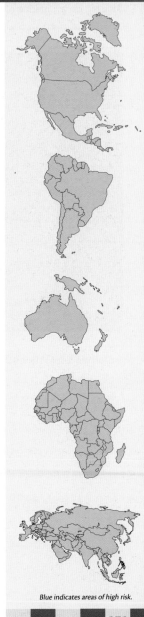

Blue indicates areas of high risk.

management may include topical cantharidin, salicylic acid, cyrotherapy, or curettage. Preventive measures are focused on avoidance of contact with lesions, which are sometimes covered with clothing or bandages to help prevent spread.

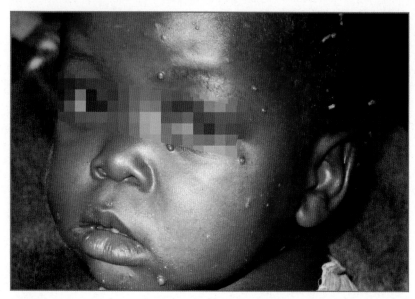

IMAGE 1

Molluscum lesions are usually asymptomatic, but can be cosmetically disagreeable.

Mumps

BACKGROUND

Mumps is caused by a moderately infectious RNA paramyxovirus that chiefly affects salivary glands, particularly the parotid. Disease occurs worldwide, and humans are the only known host. In poorly immunized populations, children aged 5 to 10 years are most affected.

PATHOPHYSIOLOGY

Transmission is via direct contact with contaminated respiratory secretions as occurs through airborne spread, from coughing or sneezing, or through fomites. Following inoculation, viral replication occurs in upper respiratory epithelium, ocular tissue, or the gastrointestinal tract. Incubation lasts 2 to 3 weeks. Subsequent viremia distributes virus throughout the body. The parotid gland is the most frequently involved tissue, but many organs can be targeted. Communicability begins several days prior to symptom onset and then continues for another week or so.

CLINICAL PRESENTATION

A nonspecific prodrome includes mild fever, anorexia, malaise, and headache. Classic mumps, accounting for approximately a third of cases, is characterized by non-suppurative swelling and tenderness of the parotid glands. The mandibular angle is distorted, and ipsilateral earlobes are sometimes displaced upward and outward. Trismus is possible. Pain may be exacerbated by citrus ingestion. On oral examination, the Stensen duct appears visibly edematous and erythematous at the meatus. Submandibular and sublingual glands may also be affected.

Some children do not manifest parotid disease. Of these, many will demonstrate only respiratory symptoms, and approximately 20% are altogether asymptomatic. A morbilliform rash may be present. Painful orchitis develops in some postpubertal boys and is a rare cause of sterility. Other potential complications include pancreatitis, hearing loss, nephritis, myocarditis, meningitis, and encephalitis. More than half of patients have evidence of central nervous

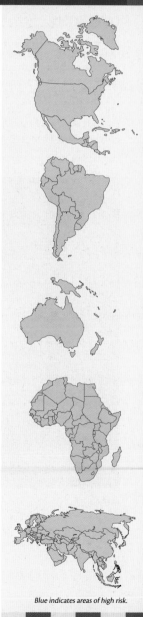

Blue indicates areas of high risk.

system infection (by way of cerebro-spinal fluid pleocytosis), but very few show related symptoms.

DIAGNOSIS

Many agents can cause parotitis, and most cases in immunized children are not due to mumps. Mumps is a leading diagnosis in those who are unimmunized. Confirmation is made by isolating virus in culture, through polymerase chain reaction, or by serology. Serum amylase may be elevated.

TREATMENT AND PREVENTION

Treatment is symptomatic and supportive. No specific antiviral therapy exists. Inpatient care is indicated for patients who suffer significant complications. Most recover without sequelae, although encephalitis can be fatal. Infection confers immunity. The best prevention is routine immunization of children. Mumps vaccine is a live attenuated virus usually given in combination with measles and rubella vaccines.

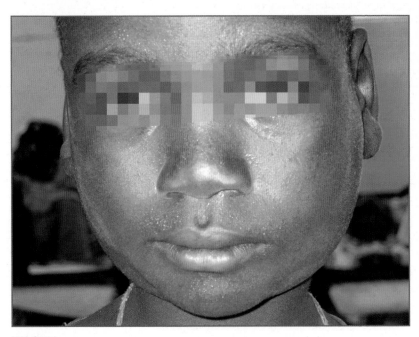

IMAGE 1

A boy with mumps. Often one parotid gland will swell and the other will follow after several days. Tenderness is usual, but overlying erythema is uncommon. Edema begins to resolve after approximately 5 days.

Noma

COMMON NAME

Cancrum oris

BACKGROUND

Noma is a devastating opportunistic, noncommunicable infection characterized by orofacial gangrene. Most cases occur in remote regions of the least developed countries, particularly in sub-Saharan Africa, Asia, and South America. Children aged 1 to 4 years are most commonly affected, and clear associations exist with extreme poverty and chronic malnutrition. Vitamin deficiency may also play a role. The true disease burden is unknown due to poor recognition and reporting behaviors, but in the late 1990s the World Health Organization estimated the incidence in children to approach 150,000. Mortality rates are as high as 80%, and those who survive are often grossly disfigured. HIV may be a predisposing factor in some children.

PATHOPHYSIOLOGY

Noma typically follows a debilitating illness (eg, measles, malaria, or diarrhea) in a stunted child. Many times the infection begins as localized gingivitis that rapidly progresses and crosses tissue planes to invade contiguous bone, muscle, subcutaneous fat, and skin. The pathogenesis is incompletely determined but may feature a complex interaction between malnutrition-induced immune deficiency and inciting environmental agents. The anaerobe *Fusobacterium necrophorum* has also been implicated. Local tissue destruction results in typical facial defects. Untreated, hematogenous dissemination is possible and significantly increases the likelihood of death.

CLINICAL PRESENTATION

Early signs include halitosis, fever, and facial edema. Gingival inflammation evolves to ulceration and extends to the lip and cheek. Lesions can be unilateral or bilateral, and grow over a matter of days to develop a black necrotic center with a well-demarcated border. Perforation of soft tissue frequently occurs. Teeth and bone often become exposed and may eventually be lost. Striking facial damage results. Survivors heal with

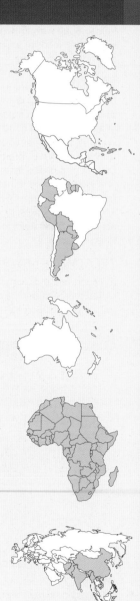

Blue indicates areas of high risk.

scarring and contractures that may leave them considerably disfigured and functionally impaired. Cosmetic injury, along with difficulties speaking and eating, leads to social isolation and psychological trauma.

DIAGNOSIS

Diagnosis of noma is entirely clinical. The history of a recent febrile illness in a malnourished child with facial swelling and foul-smelling discharge from the mouth is strongly suggestive. Culture of mucosal lesions is usually polymicrobial and unhelpful with treatment planning. Older children and adults may present with varying degrees of facial deformity in diverse stages of healing.

TREATMENT AND PREVENTION

If recognized and treated promptly, children can often be cared for successfully with antimicrobials, aggressive oral hygiene, rehydration, treatment of underlying diseases, and nutritional support. Broad-spectrum antibiotics are advocated by some, while others feel that anaerobic coverage is sufficient. Optimizing nutrition is critical but can be challenging in the context of oral cavity injury. Enteral tube feeds may be necessary. Extensive debridements are contraindicated during acute stages of disease. Reconstructive plastic surgery may be undertaken in survivors, although these services are regularly absent in many endemic areas.

Preventive measures target poverty and malnutrition. Immunization, vitamin supplementation, and education regarding good oral hygiene practices are beneficial adjunctive strategies. Intermittent examination of the oral mucosa of at-risk children is important because early antibiotic therapy is effective at preventing advanced disease.

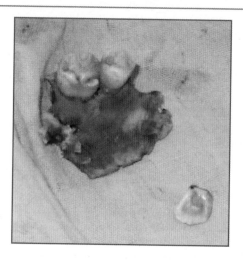

IMAGE 1

Noma is derived from the Greek word *nemo*, meaning "to devour." In sub-Saharan Africa, a field doctor was called to see a patient whose "mouth fell out." Orofacial tissue destruction had resulted in sequestration of a portion of the child's hard palate and jaw, with teeth attached. Antibiotic and nutritional therapy were administered. Fortunately, little subsequent tissue destruction occurred.

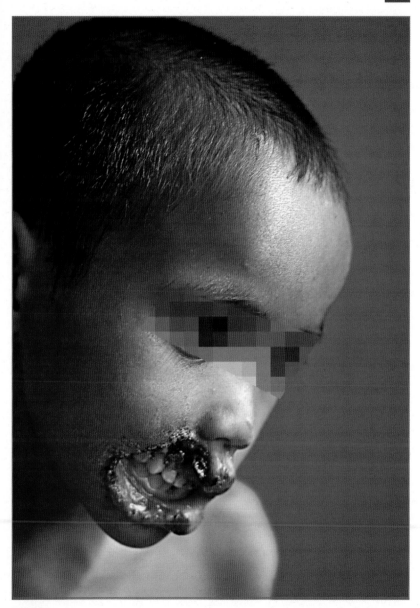

IMAGE 2

A 7-year-old boy in Laos with active noma. This stage of disease is less commonly seen by caregivers because affected children frequently live in impoverished, remote areas without access to health services. Most children die. Survivors are often shy and remain hidden, many times having been psychologically traumatized by community members who view the cosmetic damage as shameful. *Courtesy: Bryan Watt and Leila Srour.*

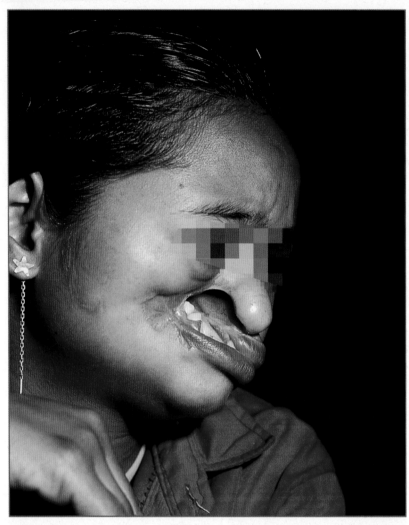

IMAGE 3

A young woman with healed noma and the first recorded survivor of the disease in Laos. She was identified by traveling physicians in a rural village reachable only by boat. There was obvious evidence of malnutrition and vitamin deficiencies among the villagers. This woman was sitting in a corner with her face to the wall. She had a hole in the side of her face and was unable to move her jaw. To eat, she pushed food through the perforation and pressed it with her fingers against her teeth. Saliva escaped from the tissue defect and her speech was limited to a whisper. She avoided social interaction, covered her face, and ate alone. Her life story was consistent with acute noma at age 4 years, surviving in veritable isolation until 18 years of age. Supported by international volunteers and donations, she underwent 3 major operations. The hole in her face has been closed, and she can now move her jaw. She eats and speaks in public and socializes more freely. *Courtesy: Bryan Watt and Leila Srour.*

Onchocerciasis

COMMON NAME

River blindness

BACKGROUND

Onchocerciasis is caused by the filarial nematode *Onchocerca volvulus* and is the world's second-leading infectious cause of blindness (following trachoma). Greater than 30 million people worldwide are infected, and more than 120 million inhabit areas that put them at high risk, including parts of Africa, Central and South America, and the Arabian Peninsula. Humans are the only definitive host. The vector, and obligatory intermediate host, is a blackfly of the genus *Simulium* that lays eggs on vegetation and rocks in rapidly flowing water bodies.

PATHOPHYSIOLOGY

The life cycle of *O volvulus* begins with the bite of an infected blackfly. Larvae enter the bloodstream via insect saliva and mature in subcutaneous tissue over a period of 6 to 12 months. Adult worms are not small: Males ultimately measure 3 to 5 cm and females grow to larger than 50 cm. Coiling of adult females produces characteristic subcutaneous nodules (onchocercomata), to which males migrate for mating. A single female produces up to several thousand eggs daily. The huge numbers of microscopic, motile microfilariae that are subsequently released cause clinical illness and play an active role in transmission. Biting blackflies take up microfilariae during a blood meal and host their maturation to infective larvae. With the next bite, a new child is infected. Microfilariae life span ranges 6 to 24 months, and adult worms may live for up to 15 years. Fortunately for travelers, transmission is relatively ineffective. Children must reside in an endemic area for an average of 2 years to acquire the parasite.

CLINICAL PRESENTATION

Firm subcutaneous nodules formed by adult worm masses are usually several centimeters in diameter and located over bony prominences. They elicit a limited immune response and produce trivial symptoms other than cosmetic disfigurement.

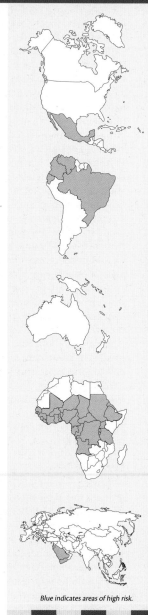

Blue indicates areas of high risk.

Most pathology of onchocerciasis stems from inflammatory and immunologic reactions to migrating and dying microfilariae, particularly in the skin and the eyes. Extent of symptomatology is related to parasite density. The incubation period ranges 3 to 36 months. Cutaneous involvement leads to intractable pruritis—some say the worst of any parasitic disease. Scratch-induced excoriations, ulcerations, and secondary infections (with regional lymphadenopathy) are common and contribute to the evolution of skin lesion morphology. Erythematous or blackened papules dominate the clinical picture in early stage dermatitis. Later signs include skin thickening, edema, lichenification, atrophy, and depigmentation. *Sowdah*, found in Yemen and Sudan, results from extreme immune hyperactivity and describes severe illness in the presence of only few microfilariae.

Ophthalmologic complications result from microfilariae presence or death in ocular tissue. Itching, erythema, photophobia, and blurred vision occur initially. Punctate keratitis, an intense inflammatory reaction, can develop into sclerosing keratitis in chronic infections. Anterior uveitis, iridocyclitis, secondary glaucoma, and optic neuritis are all possible. Progressive corneal opacification leads to blindness.

DIAGNOSIS

Diagnosis is frequently made on clinical grounds based on exposure risks and physical findings. Laboratory evaluation can be confirmatory. Direct visualization of microfilariae is achieved by microscopy of superficial, 1- to 2-mm skin snips obtained from near subcutaneous nodules. In heavy infections, motile microfilariae will be seen emerging from the snip in under an hour. For diagnosis in weaker infections with fewer microfilariae, examination of several specimens or incubation with saline may be required. Adult parasites can be found in excised nodules or identified via ultrasound. In settings with more advanced technology, ophthalmologic disease can be demonstrated on slit-lamp examination by noting free-floating microfilariae in the anterior chamber.

For suspected cases in which identification of microfilariae has been elusive, a Mazzotti diagnostic treatment test can be considered. Following a small dose of oral or topical diethylcarbamazine, a pruritic response results in infected children within hours as microfilariae die. Because severe and potentially dangerous reactions can occur, this trial should only be used in the context of light parasitic loads and when other diagnostic methods have been unsuccessful.

TREATMENT AND PREVENTION

Single-dose ivermectin is the treatment of choice, administered once or twice yearly. Ivermectin kills microfilariae over a period of days to weeks, a rate slow enough to prevent most clinically significant inflammatory reactions. Adult worms are rendered sterile with therapy, but do not die. Therefore, treatment is necessary for, at minimum, the natural life of the adult worm (up to 15 years). Toxicity of ivermectin is rare, although concerns exist regarding long-term adherence and resistance.

The Onchocerciasis Control Programme, a joint effort of the World Health Organization, the World Bank, the United Nations, and Merck & Co., Inc. distributed ivermectin and sprayed larvicide over blackfly breeding sites to control vector populations from 1974 to 2002. Thirty million people in 11 countries were treated and 600,000 cases of blindness are thought to have been prevented. Moreover, the program eliminated onchocerciasis as a public health threat in many regions; 18 million children are born in areas now free from risk of disease. Merck continues to supply ivermectin gratis through the Mectizan Donation Program, an impressive example of how private-public partnerships can effect meaningful change.

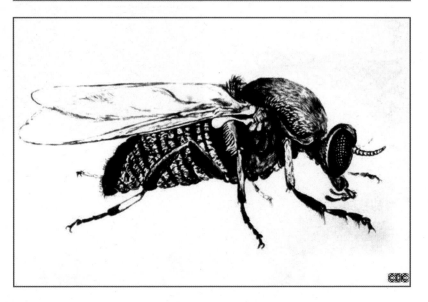

IMAGE 1

The blackfly vectors responsible for transmitting onchocerciasis have a distinctive humped thorax and are sometimes referred to as *buffalo gnats.* Clusters of 100 to 600 eggs are laid in rapidly flowing waters. The fly's life cycle then includes an aquatic larval stage. Male flies are nectar feeders; only females take blood meals from humans. *Courtesy: Centers for Disease Control and Prevention.*

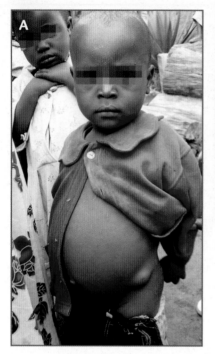

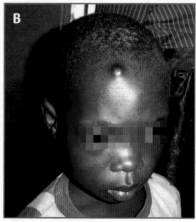

IMAGE 2A, 2B

The subcutaneous migration of adult worms is often halted by resistance encountered over bony prominences. Worms become fixed in a matte of fibrous tissue and form firm nodules measuring several centimeters. Nodules have a tendency to form near the pelvis in Africa and over the head in the Americas. *Courtesy: Mark Taylor.*

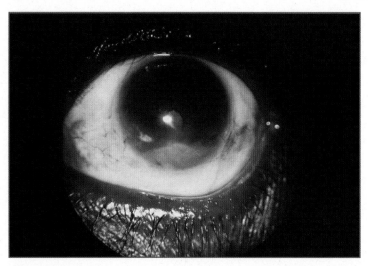

IMAGE 3

Ocular microfilaria cause an advanced inflammatory reaction in the cornea and iris. Blindness most often results from corneal scarring, chorioretinitis, or optic atrophy. Secondary cataract and glaucoma may also lead to impaired or total vision loss. *Courtesy: Larry Schwab, from* Eye Care in Developing Nations. *4th ed. London, UK: Manson Publishing Ltd; 2007.*

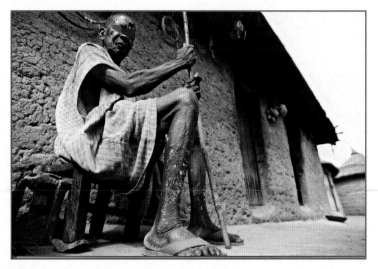

IMAGE 4

Extreme pruritis results from dermatologic infiltration of microfilariae and is a major complication of onchocerciasis. Early lesions are erythematous, papular, excoriated, and sometimes superinfected. Progression, induced in part by scratching, leads to skin blackening, lichenification, atrophy, and patchy pigment loss. *Courtesy: Larry Schwab, from* Eye Care in Developing Nations. *4th ed. London, UK: Manson Publishing Ltd; 2007.*

Pediculosis

BACKGROUND

Pediculosis affects patients of all ages and walks of life. Worldwide, hundreds of millions of cases occur each year. Lice, the organisms responsible for pediculosis, are parasites that cause dermatoses on the body (*Pediculus humanus*), scalp (*Pediculus humanus capitis*), and pubic area (*Pediculus pubis*). Among the pediatric population, the scalp is most often involved. Lice are transmitted through close contact with affected individuals or via fomites, such as hair brushes, clothing, and hats. Infestation develops in children of all socioeconomic backgrounds, particularly those living under poor conditions in which regular bathing and washing of clothes and linens is limited. Of note, body lice have been identified as vectors in epidemic typhus and trench fever outbreaks in refugee and war camps.

PATHOPHYSIOLOGY

Human beings are the exclusive hosts of lice. Adult lice are blood-sucking insects measuring 2 to 4 mm in length, are grayish-white in color, and have 6 legs that end in powerful claws. Lice typically live for 1 to 3 months, but die within 24 hours if separated from their hosts. A female louse can lay hundreds of eggs in a lifetime. These eggs, called *nits*, are laid at the base of the hair shaft and hatch within 2 weeks. Baby lice, or nymphs, are the size of a pinhead when they hatch. Maturation takes only 10 days or so, after which time adult parasites mate and complete the life cycle. Larvae and mature lice deposit feces onto the scalp or body of the host, which elicits a hypersensitivity reaction.

CLINICAL PRESENTATION

The mark of head lice infestation is the presence of nits on the shafts of the host's hair. Nits remain firmly attached to the hair even after they hatch and are not easily removed, unlike dandruff or debris. As the hair grows, nits will be seen farther distal on the hair shafts. Classically, pediculosis causes varying degrees of pruritis. Body louse infestation is associated with erythematous papular and wheal-like eruptions.

The intense scratching that is sometimes associated with pediculosis can lead to bacterial superinfection.

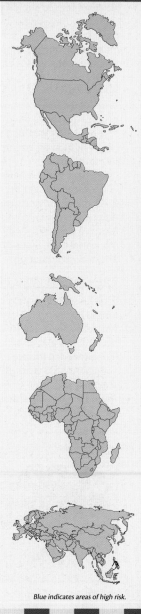

Blue indicates areas of high risk.

Impetigo of the scalp may suggest a related lice infestation. Pubic lice can be seen in high-risk sexually active adolescents and should prompt testing for other coexisting sexually transmitted infections. When seen in younger children, pubic lice should prompt consideration of possible child abuse.

DIAGNOSTIC METHODS

When head lice infestation is suspected, the hair should be parted in sections and examined thoroughly in bright light in an attempt to identify nits and moving lice. Use of a magnifying glass may be helpful. Nits are often seen in larger numbers around the nape of the neck and the ears. At times, a detection comb can assist with locating parasites. Body or pubic lice infestation is diagnosed by history and physical examination.

TREATMENT AND PREVENTION

Pediculosis is generally treated with topical insecticides. Permethrin is the treatment of choice for head lice. Malathion is also effective, but is not recommended for use in children younger than 6 years. Because of its potential toxic side effects, lindane should only be used if other treatment options have failed. An alternative

treatment of head lice includes the application of a dry-on, suffocation-based pediculicide lotion that is applied to the hair and subsequently combed out, after which the hair is dried with a hot hair drier. The hair is then shampooed several hours later. Treatment can be repeated on a weekly basis until the lice are eliminated. Body and pubic lice are most commonly treated with the application of permethrin.

Lice infestations cannot be eradicated without adequate decontamination of fomites. Every object that has touched the head or body of an affected individual must be deloused. Clothes, pillows, and sheets should be washed in hot water and dried in heat. Brushes, combs, and hair ornaments should be soaked in rubbing alcohol for approximately 1 hour and then washed in warm, soapy water.

Prevention of louse infestations is contingent on thoroughly evaluating all individuals who have had known contact with an affected individual, and treating those with evidence of disease. It is extremely important that school-aged children be educated on the importance of not sharing hats or clothing with classmates, particularly when there has been a recent outbreak of lice.

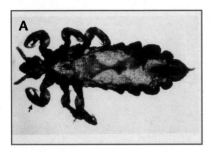
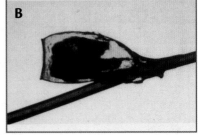

IMAGE 1A, 1B
Morphological features of a head louse (Image 1A) and a nit attached to a hair shaft (Image 1B).
Courtesy: Duke Duncan.

Pellagra

BACKGROUND

Pellagra is a systemic nutritional illness caused by cellular deficiency of the water-soluble vitamin niacin, also known as *nicotinic acid* or *Vitamin B_3*. Gasper Casal first described *pelle agra* (from the Italian, for "rough skin") in poor Spanish peasants in the mid-1700s. Primary disease results from inadequate intake of niacin or its protein precursor, the essential amino acid tryptophan, which are found in poultry, eggs, fish, red meat, whole-grain cereals, ground nuts, and vegetables. Deficiencies of micronutrients such as pyridoxine and iron that are required to convert tryptophan to niacin can also result in pellagra. Populations that suffer from chronically limited diets are at highest risk, particularly those in which niacin-poor maize or sorghum constitute regular diet staples (although this is not the case in many parts of Latin America where tortilla maize is typically washed with alkaline lime-water, a process that frees bound forms of niacin and increases its bioavailability). Primary pellagra is also found in the settings of acute nutritional crises, such as occurs in complex humanitarian emergencies, as well as in food faddists, chronic alcoholics, and those suffering from anorexia nervosa. Secondary pellagra complicates disorders that impair nutrient absorption. Some pharmaceuticals, including the antituberculosis medication isoniazid, interfere with endogenous niacin production.

PATHOPHYSIOLOGY

Dietary niacin and tryptophan are rapidly absorbed in the stomach and small intestine. They are converted to nicotinamide adenine dinucleotide and nicotinamide adenine dinucleotide phosphate, coenzymes necessary for oxidation-reduction reactions that are vital to myriad cellular functions. Elements of carbohydrate, protein, and fatty acid metabolism in multiple organs are ultimately dependent on nicotinic acid. Deficiency predominantly affects tissues with high rates of turnover (eg, skin and gastrointestinal tract) and oxidation (eg, central nervous system).

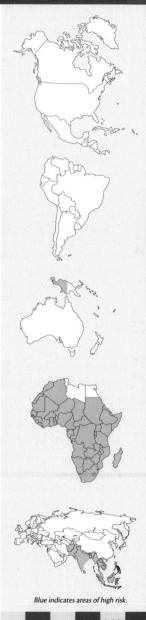

Blue indicates areas of high risk.

CLINICAL PRESENTATION

Pellagra is classically characterized by the "3 D's"—dermatitis, diarrhea, and dementia—although this triad is not always present in children. Dermatitis in pellagra involves a symmetrical, sun-exposed distribution on the face and extremities. Erythema is an early finding that may mimic severe sunburn. The rash becomes hyperpigmented, sometimes with vesiculobullous lesions that crust. Patients may complain of burning or pruritis. Eventually, skin appears scaly and thickened. Facial features can resemble the butterfly rash of systemic lupus erythematosus. The dorsum of the hands and forearms are frequently affected, and a well-marginated rim lesion follows the neckline, referred to as the *Casal necklace.*

Gastrointestinal manifestations include anorexia, nausea, emesis, abdominal pain, stomatitis, and gingivitis. Development of a swollen, beefy red tongue is not uncommon. Diarrhea results from mucosal damage. Stool may be bloody. Diarrhea-related malabsorption can aggravate baseline nutritional deficiencies.

While neurologic symptoms normally present late, they can appear early and even predate dermatitis.

Headache, irritability, anxiety, apathy, or depression give way to confusion, psychosis, and delirium. Neuritis, myelitis, and Parkinsonian symptoms are reported late in the disease course. Without treatment, coma and death may ensue, usually after a period of several years.

DIAGNOSIS

Presumptive diagnosis is based on dietary history and physical examination. Assessment of response to therapy then confirms the diagnosis. While not routinely available in most endemic regions, serum assays of niacin and its metabolites or urinary excretion studies can aid diagnosis.

TREATMENT AND PREVENTION

Oral nicotinamide administered daily is the cornerstone of treatment. Multivitamin supplementation to address other micronutrient deficiencies should also be considered.

Pellagra is prevented by ensuring a well-balanced, protein-containing diet. The recommended daily allowance of niacin ranges from 2 mg in infants to 16 mg in adolescents and 20 mg in adults (60 mg of tryptophan produces 1 mg niacin equivalent). Niacin supplements are recommended during treatment of tuberculosis with isoniazid.

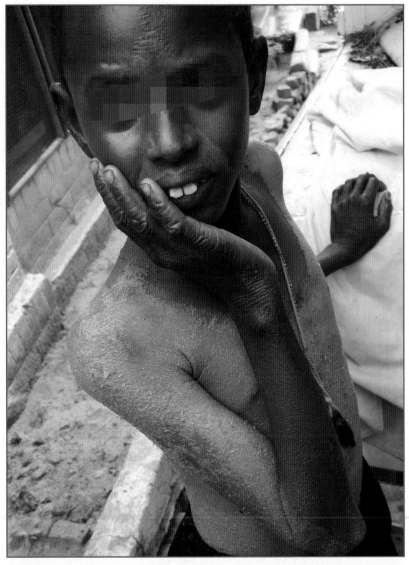

IMAGE 1
Typical photosensitive dermatitis from niacin deficiency in an adolescent presenting from an extremely remote village in sub-Saharan Africa.

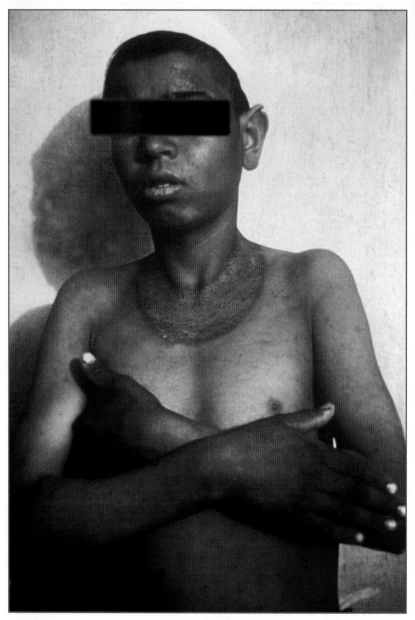

IMAGE 2
A striking example of the so-called Casal necklace. *Courtesy: Centers for Disease Control and Prevention.*

Plague

COMMON NAME

Black death

BACKGROUND

One of the oldest identifiable diseases known to man, plague remains widely distributed in the tropics and subtropics, primarily during dry and cool seasons in areas where contributing socioeconomic factors and unsanitary, rat-infested environments exist. *Yersinia pestis*, a gram-negative coccobacillus, is the causative organism. Since the 1980s a reemergence of plague has occurred often in regions that have long remained silent. Still, only a few countries on each continent carry most of the disease burden. In the 1990s, Madagascar and Tanzania accounted for nearly two-thirds of total plague cases in Africa, Brazil and Peru accounted for 80% of total cases in the Americas, and Myanmar and Vietnam accounted for most cases in Asia. In general, plague is commonest in males, adolescents, and young adults, presumably as a result of increased risk factor exposure.

PATHOPHYSIOLOGY

Essentially a disease of wild rodents, plague is spread between rodents and flea ectoparasites, particularly the species *Xenopsylla cheopis* and *Ceratophyllus fasciatus*. Transmission to humans is either by the bite of infected fleas or through handling infected hosts. During a blood meal fleas regurgitate bacteria-laden intestinal contents into skin, the mechanism for development of bubonic plague. Direct inhalation of droplets containing the organism leads to pneumonic plague. Either can spread systemically to become septicemic plague.

CLINICAL PRESENTATION

The 3 most common forms of plague are bubonic, pneumonic, and septicemic. Bubonic plague, the most common presentation of *Y pestis* infection, follows the direct inoculation of the bacteria into the skin. The site of the flea bite may be vesicular, papular, ulcerative, or unapparent. Bacteria multiply in the skin and subcutaneous tissues and travel to regional lymph nodes. Buboes, 1- to 10-cm nodes that drain the site of the

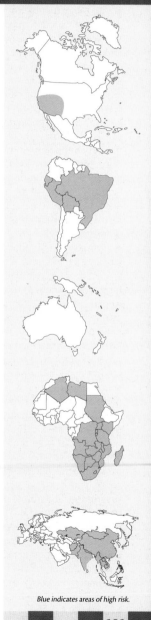

Blue indicates areas of high risk.

bite, are generally more frequent in the inguinal/femoral than axillary or cervical/submaxillary region. Following a 2- to 8-day incubation period, victims suffer from sudden onset of high fever, tachycardia, chills, weakness, headache, and prostration. Febrile seizures in children are common. Enlarged lymph nodes become inflamed and tender, and the surrounding skin may become discolored or purpuric. Hematogenous spread can lead to bacteremia, septicemia, secondary pneumonia (particularly of bilateral lower lobes), and organ failure. Untreated, mortality rates approach 50%. Although uncommon, a more favorable clinical course can occur. A few patients spontaneously recover even without specific antimicrobial therapy.

Primary pneumonic plague is acquired by inhaling infective aerosolized droplets released from the feces or respiratory tract of infected humans or animals. Rapid and robust multiplication of bacteria in the lung parenchyma results in bacteremia. Two to 3 days after exposure, a sudden onset of productive cough (with frothy, blood-tinged, hemorrhagic, or purulent sputum) is accompanied by fever, chest pain, dyspnea, and hypoxia. Diarrhea, agitation, prostration, and coma may occur. Untreated, the pneumonia becomes overwhelming, and mortality approaches 100%.

Septicemic plague occurs when severe endotoxemia, hypotension, prostration, abdominal pain, nausea, vomiting, diarrhea, and multiple organ failure occur without identifiable lymphadenopathy. Presumably, this results from a high-density bacteremia with endotoxin release resulting in disseminated intravascular coagulation and shock. Mortality, even with treatment, exceeds 30%.

Pharyngitis and meningitis are uncommon manifestations of *Y pestis* infection, often after inadequate treatment of the more common disease entities.

DIAGNOSIS

Diagnostic aspiration of the infected lymph nodes, subcutaneous tissues, or purulent exudates usually yields an ovoid, nonmotile coccobacilli that characteristically stains in a "safety-pin" fashion, with accumulation of stain at both poles. In settings with limited diagnostic services, the gram stain diagnosis may be the only reliable laboratory confirmation method available. Peripheral leukocytosis occurs frequently with the presence of band forms and toxic granulations. Occasionally the bacillus is visible on peripheral blood smear. Approximately 25% of untreated victims with bubonic plague have positive blood cultures. Chest radiography in pneumonic plague initially demonstrates a unilateral infiltrate that quickly progresses to patchy, diffuse, and bilateral pneumonia. Polymerase chain reaction, immunofluorescence staining, and hemaglutination testing for anti-F1 antigen titers may assist with confirmation of diagnosis.

TREATMENT AND PREVENTION

Appropriate antibiotic therapy reduces bubonic plague mortality rates to 5% to 15%. Effective therapy includes streptomycin, doxycycline, tetracycline hydrochloride, gentamicin, ciprofloxacin, and chloramphenicol. Chloramphenicol remains the most effective antimicrobial for plague meningitis. Supportive care, with meticulous attention to fluid management, is essential. Contact and respiratory precautions using appropriate personal protective equipment is important for health care workers.

Preventing human plague is achieved by implementing comprehensive public health programs that include surveillance, diagnosis, education, and training programs for the general public and health care workers, specifically regarding vector control and avoidance. Pesticides should be used when necessary, and the handling of dead rodents is to be avoided.

A plague vaccine exists that likely reduces the incidence and severity of bubonic plague. Its effect against pneumonic plague is unclear. Immunization is typically reserved for those working directly with *Y pestis* or those engaged in field activities in areas of active disease. Postexposure prophylaxis with trimethoprim-sulfamethoxazole or doxycycline is recommended within 7 days of exposure for persons with direct, close contact with a pneumonic plague patient, or those exposed to a possibly contaminated aerosol.

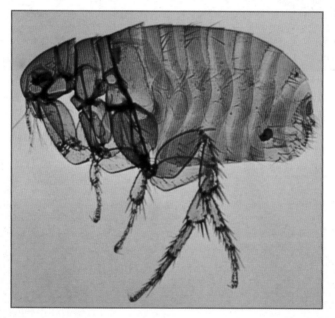

IMAGE 1

The female *Xenopsylla cheopis flea*, sometimes known as the *oriental rat flea*, transmits *Yersina pestis. Courtesy: World Health Organization.*

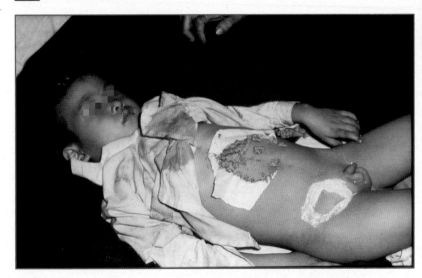

IMAGE 2

A child presented with a tender groin bubo, fever, and weakness. The parent had placed a limelike gritty substance around the bubo to limit its growth, a pasty substance on the abdomen with Chinese writings as petitions to gods versed in medicine, and onion flacks in the scalp hair to control fever. The child survived but developed clinical sepsis and prolonged febrile seizures. *Courtesy: Frederick M. Burkle Jr.*

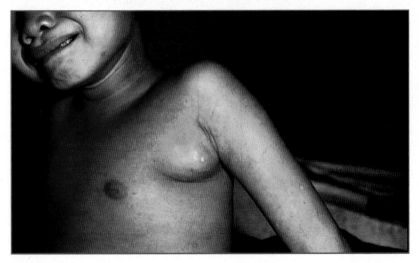

IMAGE 3

This 8-year-old female was the sentinel case of a plague epidemic. An axillary bubo was aspirated and revealed sheets of bipolar coccobacilli. The lymph node tissue was destroyed by the infectious process. She recovered well with oral antibiotics but regression and closure of the node took several months to heal. *Courtesy: Frederick M. Burkle Jr.*

Poliomyelitis

COMMON NAME

Infantile paralysis

BACKGROUND

Poliomyelitis is a highly contagious viral illness that may result in paralysis and death. Infections with polioviruses occur only in humans and are more common in infants and young children. While disease is most frequent during the summer and fall seasons in temperate zones, seasonal variation is less obvious in tropical climates. A major international eradication initiative, currently in progress, has dramatically reduced the number of wild-type cases worldwide to less than 1,500. Four endemic countries remain: Afghanistan, India, Nigeria, and Pakistan. The few cases that continue to emerge in industrialized countries are largely vaccine-associated paralytic poliomyelitis resulting from administration of the oral poliovirus vaccine.

PATHOPHYSIOLOGY

Poliomyelitis results primarily from fecal-oral transmission of poliovirus, a small RNA enterovirus. The virus multiplies in the pharynx and intestines and is shed in stool. Children spontaneously clear the virus, harbor it as an asymptomatic carrier, or suffer subsequent viremia and central nervous system (CNS) infection. Poliovirus can spread along motor nerve fibers and destroy them at a frighteningly brisk pace. Three serotypes exist. Infection with one type does not protect against others, but lifelong immunity is conferred to the infecting strain. Poliovirus type 1 causes most paralytic cases.

CLINICAL PRESENTATION

More than 90% of infections are asymptomatic and less than 1% result in paralysis. Symptoms associated with viremia follow an incubation period of 6 to 20 days. Nonspecific malaise, fever, and pharyngitis are common. Central nervous system involvement leads to clinical pictures suggestive of aseptic meningitis or encephalitis. Paralytic polio is typically classified as spinal, bulbar, or bulbospinal. Spinal polio is characterized by rapid and asymmetrical acute flaccid paralysis with limb areflexia. Permanency of disability is determined

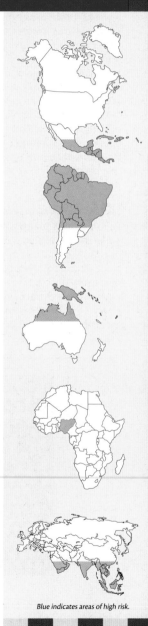

Blue indicates areas of high risk.

by the degree of neuronal damage. Some cells may be only temporarily injured and regain function after 4 to 6 weeks. Death is rare. Bulbar polio, in which virus invades the brain stem, is less common. Limb involvement is minimal in this form but mortality is high due to vasomotor disturbances including autonomic dysfunction, dysphagia, hypotension, and respiratory failure. Bulbospinal polio has elements of both spinal and bulbar disease. Postpoliomyelitis syndrome refers to a constellation of neuromuscular symptoms that occurs as long as 30 years after primary infection.

DIAGNOSIS

Poliomyelitis should be suspected in children who live in endemic regions or nearby countries and present with acute flaccid paralysis in the absence of sensory or cognitive loss. Laboratory diagnosis is by viral culture from stool, pharynx, or cerebrospinal fluid (CSF). Yield is greatest early in the disease course. In CNS disease, CSF analysis usually reveals mild pleocytosis with a lymphocytic predominance.

TREATMENT AND PREVENTION

Treatment is supportive. No antiviral agent against poliovirus exists. Intensive care including mechanical ventilation may be required in patients with severe illness. Muscle paresis and paralysis can result in long-term skeletal and muscular deformities. Physical rehabilitation is essential. Braces and corrective shoes may be required. In some cases, surgical intervention is necessary.

Poliomyelitis is entirely preventable by proper immunization. Oral (live-attenuated) and intramuscular (inactivated) forms of poliovirus vaccine are available. The inactivated preparation is preferred in high-income countries to decrease the risk of vaccine-associated disease, but oral polio vaccine remains the vaccine of choice in most developing countries. Oral polio vaccine is inexpensive, easy to administer, and confers excellent immunity in the intestine—critical features for achieving global eradicaton.

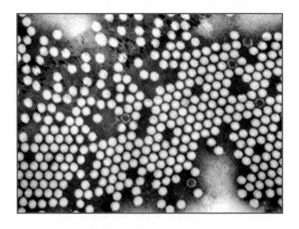

IMAGE 1

Structurally, poliovirus is strikingly simple. It consists of a short, single-strand of RNA enclosed in a non-enveloped icosahedral protein capsid. *Courtesy: Centers for Disease Control and Prevention/Fred Murphy and Sylvia Whitfield.*

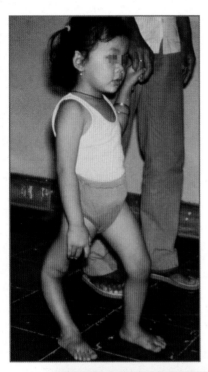

IMAGE 2
A child's limb deformity marks the permanent sequella of paralytic polio. The virus crippled thousands of children each year until the late 1950s, when the first polio vaccine was introduced. Poliomyelitis remains a scourge in select countries. Most cases in 2008 occurred in Nigeria and India. *Courtesy: Centers for Disease Control and Prevention.*

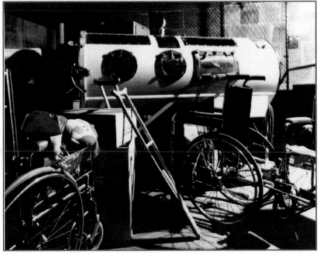

IMAGE 3
A haunting image depicts therapeutic tools associated with childhood polio. Iron lungs were commonly used for respiratory support in the 1940s and 1950s. *Courtesy: Centers for Disease Control and Prevention/Meredith Hickson.*

Poststreptococcal Glomerulonephritis

BACKGROUND

Acute poststreptococcal glomerulonephritis (APSGN) is a sequela of group A streptococcal (GAS) pharyngeal or skin infection. Distribution is worldwide, although prevalence is greatest in tropical regions where cutaneous infections are common. Peak incidence is in children aged 2 to 6 years. Disease is usually sporadic but can occur in epidemics.

PATHOPHYSIOLOGY

Group A streptococcal strains that possess certain "M" types of protein are nephritogenic. Acute poststreptococcal glomerulonephritis is likely an immune-mediated disorder in which antigen-antibody complexes are deposited at the glomerular basement membrane. An alternate hypothesis suggests antigenic mimicry produces autoantibodies that cross-react with and damage glomerular tissue. Symptoms follow pharyngitis by 10 days or so and skin infection by approximately 3 weeks. Although the most likely cause of reactive renal disease is preceding GAS infection, other bacterial agents have also been implicated in post-infectious nephritis.

CLINICAL PRESENTATION

Disease is characterized by abrupt onset of oliguria and fluid retention. Periorbital and dependent edema are common. Respiratory symptoms, including cough, dyspnea, and orthopnea, may develop secondary to pulmonary congestion. Microscopic hematuria is present in nearly all children, and up to half suffer from gross hematuria. Urine generally becomes dark in color. Hypertension is a frequent complication, sometimes with associated headache, vomiting, and even encephalopathy in severe cases.

DIAGNOSIS

Clinical diagnosis is supported by urinalysis (eg, hematuria, red blood cell casts, and occasionally proteinuria) and evidence of recent GAS infection (eg, positive pharyngeal culture or streptococcal serologies). Complement levels, if measured, are uniformly

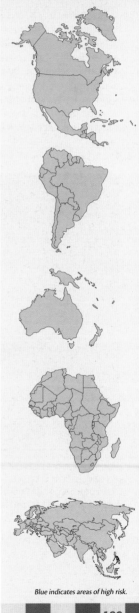

Blue indicates areas of high risk.

depressed. A minority of patients have mild renal failure with resultant electrolyte disturbances.

TREATMENT AND PREVENTION

Management of children with APSGN is largely supportive and aimed at correction of abnormalities associated with fluid retention, hypertension, and acute renal insufficiency. Fluid and salt restriction, sometimes with loop diuretic therapy, is often prescribed. Prognosis is excellent. Complete recovery occurs in more than 95% of patients. Long-standing glomerulonephritis, chronic renal failure, and need for dialysis are rare.

Unlike acute rheumatic fever (another GAS sequela), early treatment of GAS infections does not prevent progression to glomerulonephritis. Nor do antibiotics hasten the resolution of APSGN symptoms. Still, patients with APSGN should be treated with penicillin once diagnosed to prevent spread of nephritogenic strains.

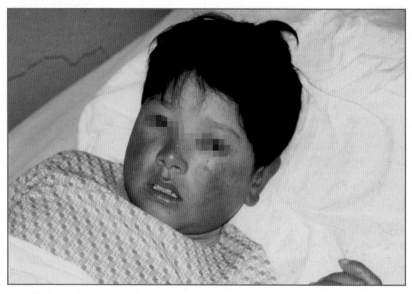

IMAGE 1

A young patient in Ecuador suffers from a common disease complex: scabies, followed by group A streptococcus superinfection, followed by poststreptococcal glomerulonephritis. The boy is hypertensive and has mild facial edema.

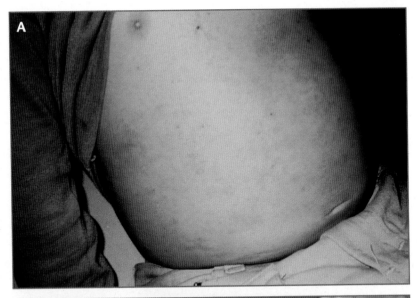

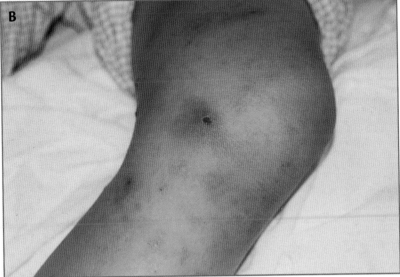

IMAGE 2A, 2B
The boy (in Image 1) also has a swollen trunk and limbs. He has healing cutaneous lesions.

Pyomyositis, Tropical

BACKGROUND

Tropical pyomyositis is a suppurative bacterial infection of skeletal muscles found worldwide but occuring primarily in tropical regions. Boys are more commonly affected, and the peak incidence occurs between the ages of 5 to 9 years. Immunocompromised states increase the risk of disease.

PATHOPHYSIOLOGY

While the exact pathophysiology remains unknown, *Staphylococcus aureus* (95%) is by far the most frequently identified etiologic agent. Minor trauma is occasionally recalled, presumably leading to muscle injury that predisposes to infection. Abscesses commonly develop, often multiple, and patients may be measurably bacteremic. Systemic spread can occur with the development of full-blown sepsis.

CLINICAL PRESENTATION

Onset is usually insidious, with pain and swelling of the involved muscle. Larger muscle groups of the lower extremities, particularly the quadriceps, hamstrings, and gluteals, are affected most frequently. The average interval between symptom onset and presentation is 3 weeks. Initially, pain is crampy and accompanied by low-grade fever. As the disease progresses, local inflammation increases. Warmth, edema, erythema, and fluctuance signal underlying abscess formation. Patients presenting in the early invasive stage demonstrate a woody, tender swelling of the involved muscles, whereas those in the invasive stage demonstrate warm, erythematous edema with extreme tenderness. In cases where abscesses are deep-seated, local signs of inflammation may be absent. Primary involvement of the psoas muscle may present with hip flexion and external rotation. Curiously, regional lymph node enlargement is many times absent. Some children run a slow, chronic course, whereas others suffer from fulminant disease characterized by the presence of toxemia and disseminated intravascular coagulation.

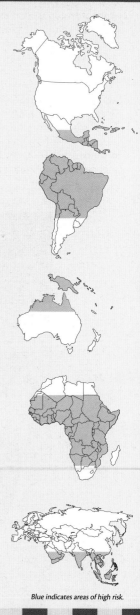

Blue indicates areas of high risk.

DIAGNOSIS

Experienced clinicians working in endemic regions often make clinical diagnoses. Ultrasound examination of the affected muscle group can be helpful. Features include diffuse muscular infiltration or well-defined abscesses. Magnetic resonance imaging may detect infection earlier, but is rarely available in most resource-limited settings. Cultures of purulent material or blood can confirm the diagnosis and assist in identification of the inciting organism. Other laboratory findings such as left-shifted leukocytosis and elevated inflammatory markers (eg, erythrocyte sedimentation rate, C-reactive protein) can be helpful but are nonspecific.

TREATMENT AND PREVENTION

Oral anti-staphylococcal antibiotic therapy can arrest disease progression in early stages. In more advanced cases, incision and drainage of pus collections, when they exist, is imperative. Parenteral antibiotics are also indicated for invasive disease. Prevention is difficult. Early recognition and prompt treatment is of paramount importance.

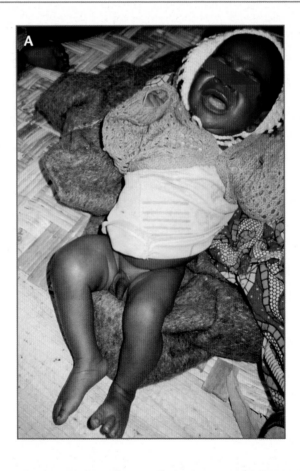

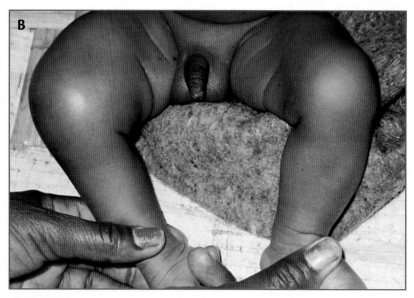

IMAGE 1A, 1B

Tropical pyomyositis can be a frustrating condition to manage. The muscle of this young Angolan's thigh was obviously infected but without a circumscribed, drainable pus collection.

Rabies

BACKGROUND

Rabies is a zoonosis caused by an RNA *Lyssavirus*
and transmitted via saliva of infected mammals.
The disease is endemic everywhere, except on a few
islands including Australia, New Zealand, Hawaii, and
Antarctica. Despite the existence of an effective vaccine, more than 50,000 people die from rabies each
year, primarily in rural Asia and Africa. Virtually all
cases in less developed countries result from contact
with rabid canines. Children are at increased risk
because they tend to spend more time near dogs and
are more likely to suffer bites to the face and neck,
which represent particularly infectious exposures. In
industrialized countries, wild animals such as bats,
skunks, raccoons, foxes, and coyotes are the most
common reservoirs and sources of infection. Domestic
dogs, cats, and ferrets have also been implicated. Virus
is transmitted in 15% to 40% of attacks from rabid
animals.

PATHOPHYSIOLOGY

Affected canines demonstrate 1 of 2 phenotypes. Some
dogs are completely mad, rush aimlessly, and bite
indiscriminately (objects as well as people). In others,
illness manifests as so-called dumb rabies, in which
lethargy and paralysis predominate. Viral loads are high
in saliva and virus is spread during a bite or scratch.
Less frequently, transmission occurs without dermal compromise by saliva contamination of mucous
membranes.

The incubation period in humans is typically 3 to
12 weeks, but may be as long as 1 year. In general, bites
on the extremities result in longer incubations than
those on the head and neck because virus particles
take longer to migrate through peripheral axons to the
central nervous system (CNS). After replication, virus
disseminates systemically. While the exact mechanism
by which rabies induces neurotoxicity is poorly understood, it is well established that viral effects on neural
tissue are ultimately fatal. Mortality may also result
from myocarditis-induced arrhythmias or congestive
heart failure.

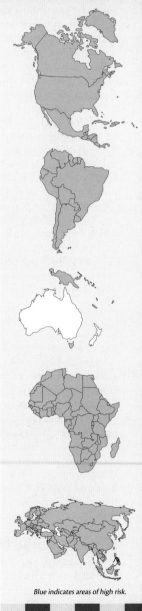

Blue indicates areas of high risk.

207

CLINICAL PRESENTATION

Disease is heralded in many children by a prodrome of headache, fever, and subtle mental status changes. As illness progresses, symptoms take the form of either "furious" or "paralytic" rabies.

Eighty percent of cases are of the furious variety, with signs of severe encephalitis. Painful muscle spasms are triggered in response to physical, aural, and olfactory stimuli. In later stages, throat spasms and intense pain on swallowing cause hydrophobia, an excited panic at the prospect of consuming fluid. Delirium, hallucinations, behavior changes, autonomic dysfunction, and seizures are possible. Paralytic rabies is less common and is characterized by an ascending flaccid paralysis in which symptoms largely reflect spinal cord involvement.

Both forms of disease eventually lead to paralysis and coma 2 to 14 days after onset of symptoms. Death follows.

DIAGNOSIS

Rabies must be considered in a child with progressive encephalopathy and a history of an animal bite or scratch. However, no symptoms are pathognomonic. When resources permit, rabies can be diagnosed by polymerase chain reaction of infected body fluids (saliva, tears, urine, or cerebrospinal fluid), serology, or immunofluorescence of skin biopsy specimens. If necessary, definitive diagnosis is made postmortem by direct fluorescent antibody evaluation of CNS tissue.

TREATMENT AND PREVENTION

In most settings, rabies is invariably fatal once clinical signs appear.

Following a high-risk exposure, it is critical to rapidly provide local wound care and work toward imparting passive and active immunity. Bite or scratch wounds from potentially rabid animals should be copiously irrigated and cleansed with soap and iodine. Necrotic tissue is to be excised. Rabies postexposure prophylaxis (PEP) is extremely effective and should be initiated as soon as possible. Postexposure prophylaxis involves wound infiltration with rabies immune globulin and administration of multiple doses of intramuscular rabies vaccine. Several rabies PEP vaccination schedules exist, most using a 4- or 5-dose regimen. Antibiotics and tetanus prophylaxis may be required in some children.

After a low-risk exposure (eg, by a healthy domesticated pet), PEP may be temporarily deferred while the animal is confined and closely monitored. An infectious animal will become ill and die within a 10-day observation period. In some cases, authorities are uncomfortable waiting, and the animal is sacrificed to permit CNS tissue evaluation. Bat bite lesions are often subclinical. As such, PEP should be strongly considered following possible bat contact unless there is certainty that a bite, scratch, or mucous membrane exposure did not occur. Postexposure prophylaxis is rarely, if ever, indicated following rodent exposure.

The key to preventing human rabies in less developed countries is targeting canine disease through animal vaccination programs and population control. Pre-exposure prophylaxis with rabies vaccine is recommended for children at increased risk, including those with occupational hazards and travelers to some enzootic countries.

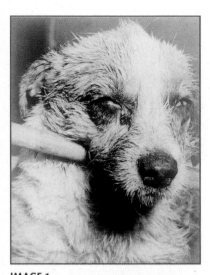

IMAGE 1

Dumb rabies in dogs is characterized by lethargy, discoordination, and paralysis. Drooling results from paralysis of throat and jaw muscles. *Courtesy: Centers for Disease Control and Prevention/Barbara Andrews.*

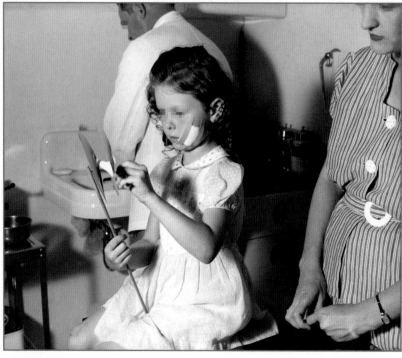

IMAGE 2

A young girl's facial wound is cleansed by her physician following a bite by a suspected rabid animal. She will also receive rabies postexposure prophylaxis (PEP). In the United States, high-risk exposures lead to administration of PEP to approximately 40,000 people each year. Unfortunately, the regimen is not readily available in parts of many less developed countries, where most rabies deaths now occur. *Courtesy: Centers for Disease Control and Prevention.*

Rickets

COMMON NAME

Rachitis

BACKGROUND

Rickets is a disease of deficient bone mineralization. Descriptions of affected European children date back to the 1600s, but the causal relationships with polluted environments and insufficient diet were not recognized for another several hundred years. Incidence is highest in children aged 6 to 24 months.

Vitamin D deficiency is the most common etiology. Because photochemical reactions in the skin catalyzed by ultraviolet light produce active vitamin D, children with limited sun exposure are at risk. This includes those living in communities where air quality is poor, those whose cultural dress covers most of the body, and those who live beyond the 37th parallel (north or south). Darkly pigmented individuals constitute another high-risk group because their skin absorbs less sunlight.

Nutritional deficiencies also lead to rickets. Breast milk is low in vitamin D, and exclusively breastfed infants require supplementation. In older children, rickets stems from inadequate intake of calcium and, sometimes, phosphorous.

Less frequently, rickets is a consequence of genetic causes (eg, vitamin D-dependent rickets types 1 and 2), malabsorption, or chronic renal disease.

PATHOPHYSIOLOGY

Bone is formed by osteoblast-mediated construction of osteoid (the bony "matrix") and subsequent mineralization (incorporation of calcium, phosphorous, and other minerals into the osteoid scaffold). Flawed osteoid production is called *osteopenia. Rickets,* or *osteomalacia,* refers to insufficient mineralization.

Vitamin D is responsible for regulating serum levels of calcium and phosphorous, which are central to processes of bone mineralization and resorption. The first step in the endogenous synthesis of vitamin D occurs in the epidermis, where 7-dehydrocholesterol is converted to vitamin D_3 in the presence of sunlight. Vitamin D_3 is hydroxylated once in the liver and again

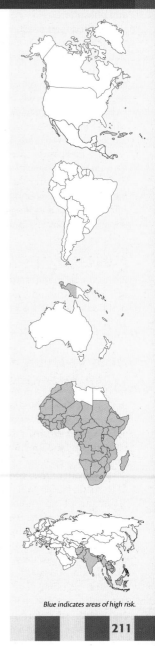

Blue indicates areas of high risk.

in the kidneys to produce calcitriol, the bioactive form of vitamin D that stimulates intestinal absorption of calcium and phosphorous.

Fortified food products constitute the richest sources of dietary vitamin D. Natural sources include fish oils, egg yolks, and certain mushrooms. Children with sufficient sun exposure do not require high quantities of nutritional vitamin D but must have adequate calcium intake. Low serum calcium levels induce parathyroid hormone secretion, which signals osteoclasts to resorb (demineralize) bone. Mineralizing cartilage is also affected in rickets, particularly at sites of rapid growth and remodeling such as long bone epiphyses and metaphyses, and at costochondral junctions.

CLINICAL PRESENTATION

Early clinical manifestations include craniotabes (thinning and softening of the skull, which may then "pop" on deep palpation), head asymmetry, frontal bossing, and delayed closure of the anterior fontanel. Tooth eruption may be late, with abnormal formation of enamel and increased propensity for dental caries. *Rachitic rosary* refers to palpable and sometimes visible bony protuberances at the anterior aspects of ribs formed by enlargement of costochondral junctions. As rickets progresses, a pigeon chest irregularity develops, oftentimes with appearance of Harrison groove (a horizontal crease across the inferior thorax created from inward tension of the diaphragm on a softened rib cage). Children may present with motor delays and low tone due to muscle weakness. Following ambulation, classic limb abnormalities manifest including genu varum (leg bowing), genu valgum (knock knees), and windswept deformities (genu varum of one leg and valgum of the other). Fraying, widening, or cupping at the metaphysis of long bones may be evident on examination (as wrist flaring) or radiograph. Rickets imposes an increased risk of fractures, lordosis, kyphosis, and scoliosis.

DIAGNOSIS

Clinical diagnosis can be made following a thorough history of sun exposure and diet in the context of signs and symptoms of hypocalcemia. Family history of rickets or bone deformities may be supportive. Biochemical disturbances depend on the mechanism of disease. In vitamin D deficiency, serum 25-hydroxyvitamin D, calcium, and phosphorous levels are low; parathyroid hormone, alkaline phosphatase, and urinary phosphorous are generally elevated. In rickets caused by poor calcium intake, 25-hydroxyvitamin D and phosphorus levels are many times normal; 1,25-dihydroxyvitamin D is elevated; and serum calcium is low.

TREATMENT AND PREVENTION

Vitamin D–deficient rickets is treated with oral or intramuscular replacement, usually in the form of ergocalciferol. Once levels have normalized, continued adequate maintenance intake is critical. In children with nutritional deficiencies, calcium supplementation is important and more effective than vitamin D supplementation alone. While augmenting ultraviolet light exposure may play a role in rickets management, vitamin D and calcium supplementation remain the most reliable methods of treatment.

With proper therapy, prognosis for rickets related to malnutrition is good. Most children with mild-to-moderate limb abnormalities show radiographic improvement in weeks and clinical improvement within 6 months. Those with more severe skeletal abnormalities may have persistent defects and benefit from splinting or orthopedic surgery, when available.

Preventive measures include ensuring ample time in the sun, while taking care to prevent sunburn. However, quantifying optimal exposure time is difficult because it is contingent on latitude, season, time of day, skin pigmentation, extent of clothing, and air quality. As little as 30 to 60 minutes weekly may be sufficient. Dark-skinned children require longer exposure times. In many countries, exclusively breastfed infants are empirically supplemented with vitamin D.

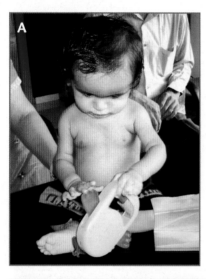

IMAGE 1A, 1B
Frontal bossing and widened wrist epiphyses suggest chronic and severe rickets. *Courtesy: Ashok Kapse.*

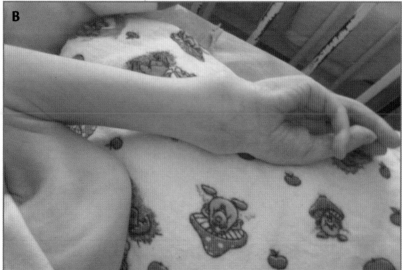

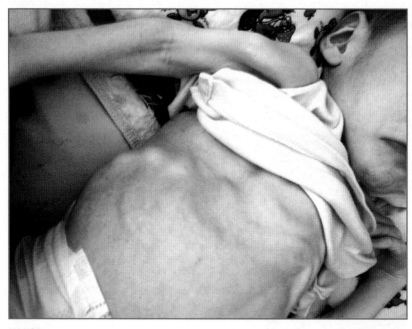

IMAGE 2
Rickets can be a clue to neglect, abuse, or malnutrition. Rachitic rosary was noted in this institutionalized orphan in Eastern Europe, who likely suffered from both limited sun exposure and dietary deficiencies.

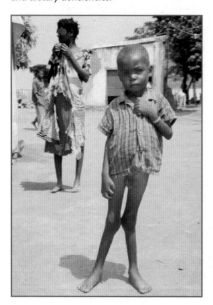

IMAGE 3
Characteristic rickets-associated genu valgum in rural Angola.

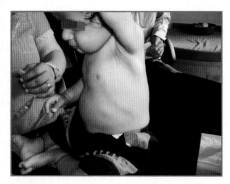

IMAGE 4

Harrison groove in a young Asian child. *Courtesy: Ashok Kapse.*

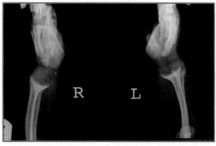

IMAGE 5

Radiographic deformities in rickets, demonstrating cupping, fraying, and widening of the distal radius and humerus. *Courtesy: Ashok Kapse.*

Scabies

COMMON NAMES

Seven-year itch

BACKGROUND

Scabies is an exceptionally pruritic eruption caused by the cosmopolitan ectoparasite *Sarcoptes scabiei* (subspecies *hominis*). The global disease burden exceeds 300 million cases annually. Poverty, overcrowding, and immunosuppression are important predisposing factors. *S scabiei* infestation is exclusive of humans. Dogs and cats can transmit related mites, which cause similar but comparatively minor and short-lived symptoms.

PATHOPHYSIOLOGY

Transmission is by close proximity to affected persons or fomites, especially clothing or bedding, on which mites can survive for up to 3 days. At least 5 minutes is thought to be necessary for effective migration to a new host, so transient contact of limited duration puts one at minimal risk. Mites are incapable of flying or jumping from person to person.

New infections are initiated only by gravid females that dig into the superficial epidermis and create a single burrow. Tunneling is directionless and occurs at a rate of several millimeters daily. Eggs and feces, referred to as *scybalum*, are deposited in mite paths and contribute to a hypersensitivity response that triggers the intractable itch. Larvae hatch in 48 hours, climb from the burrow, molt, and mature. Adults mate on the skin surface, after which males die and females begin again the process of excavation. Mite life span is less than 2 months.

CLINICAL PRESENTATION

An incubation of 4 to 6 weeks occurs with primary infection, corresponding to the period in which an allergic reaction develops to mite saliva, eggs, and feces. On repeat exposures, after sensitization has occurred, symptoms appear in only a few days.

Papules, vesicles, or pustules often develop at the site of inoculation. The characteristic burrow is a gray or white serpiginous thread that ultimately extends more than a centimeter. Scybala are sometimes visible

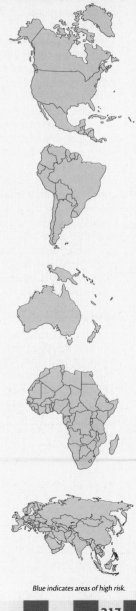

Blue indicates areas of high risk.

as dark areas within individual tracts, and the tunnel terminus may also have a darkened spot that represents the female mite (assuming she has not yet been "scratched out"). Mites tend to burrow where there are few sebaceous glands and a thin stratum corneum, most notably the interdigital spaces, axillary folds, anterior wrists, buttocks, genitalia, and nipple region. Lesions in younger children are commonly also found on the face, head, and neck. Infants who crawl are affected on the palms and soles. Pruritis can be intense and is generally worse at night. With persistent scratching, burrows are often obliterated and eczematized. Excoriated areas are susceptible to bacterial superinfection.

Norwegian, or "crusted," scabies is a severe form that affects immunocompromised children. Lesions are generalized with papules, vesicles, crusts, and thick white-gray plaques with variable grades of fissuring.

DIAGNOSIS

Diagnosis is confirmed by demonstration of mites, eggs, or feces in skin scrapings from sites with suggestive lesions. Specimens are most fruitful when collected from the terminal portion of a burrow and best viewed with an added drop of mineral oil. Although simple to perform, microscopic confirmation is not necessary when classic symptoms and skin lesions are present. HIV testing is recommended when Norwegian scabies is manifest.

TREATMENT AND PREVENTION

Topical scabicides such as permethrin 5% or benzyl benzoate are treatments of choice. These are applied to the entire body (except face and mucous membranes) for the prescribed period and then washed off. Second applications, after 1 week, are sometimes indicated. A single dose of oral ivermectin is also effective, but its use is reserved for refractory disease or Norwegian scabies. In all cases, strongly consider simultaneously treating the entire family and laundering clothing and bedding in hot or boiling water. Potentially infected items that are non-washable should be sealed in a plastic bag for 4 days. Warn patients that pruritis may persist for 1 to 2 weeks following therapy and, therefore, does not represent treatment failure. Oral antihistamines, calamine lotion, or topical steroids can be used for symptomatic relief. Avoidance of infected individuals and materials is the cornerstone of prevention.

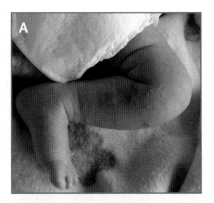

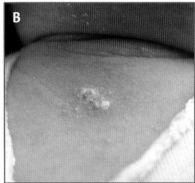

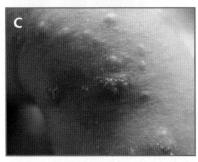

IMAGE 1A–1C

Scabies in a 5-week-old infant. Papules, vesicles, and pustules can occur without visible burrows (Image 1A). Extension of disease to chest and neck was complicated by crusting (Image 1B). A detailed view of lesions shows typical morphology (Image 1C). *Courtesy: Javier Santisteban-Ponce.*

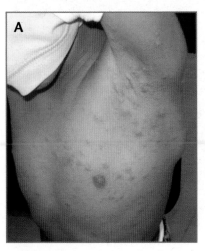

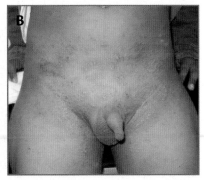

IMAGE 2A, 2B

A young boy with scabies in South America. *Sarcoptes scabiei* mites have 8 legs and are approximately 400 µm long, just barely visible to the naked eye. *Courtesy: Javier Santisteban-Ponce.*

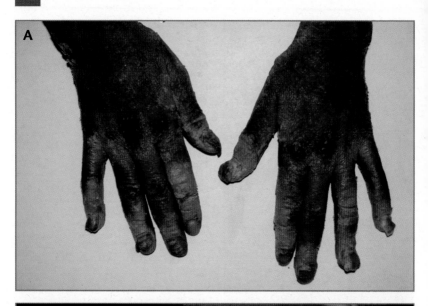

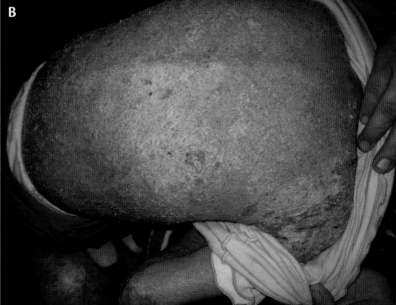

IMAGE 3A, 3B

Norwegian scabies in an HIV-infected boy in sub-Saharan Africa (Image 3A) and a child in Peru (Image 3B). Whereas typical scabies infestations are usually characterized by 10 to 20 mites, crusted scabies often has in excess of several hundred parasites and is considerably more contagious. *Courtesy: Elizabeth Dufort and Francsico Bravo.*

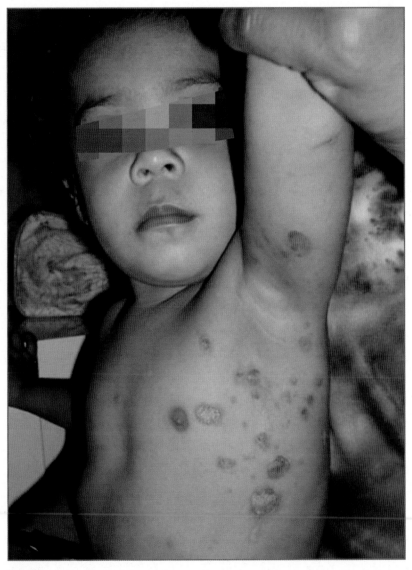

IMAGE 4

Bacterial superinfections can complicate scabies. In these cases, antibiotic treatment is often initiated several days prior to topical scabicides. *Courtesy: Stephanie Doniger.*

Schistosomiasis

COMMON NAMES

Bilharzia, Clam digger's itch, Katayama fever,
Swimmer's itch

BACKGROUND

Schistosomiasis is a visceral parasitic disease transmitted to children by contact with free-living larvae in freshwater bodies. The causative agent is 1 of 5 species of fluke: *Schistosoma haematobium* primarily affects the genitourinary tract while *Schistosoma mansoni*, *Schistosoma intercalatum*, *Schistosoma japonicum*, and *Schistosoma mekongi* typically target the intestines and liver. The most important species in terms of disease burden are *S haematobium*, *S mansoni*, and *S japonicum*. Nearly 800 million people are at risk of schistosomiasis and more than 200 million people are infected across 70 countries in tropical and subtropical Africa, South America, the Middle East, East Asia, and the Philippines. Prevalence rates in endemic regions may exceed 50%. Humans are the main reservoir and definitive host. Aquatic snails (or amphibious snails in the case of *S japonicum*) of various species host an obligatory intermediate form of the parasite, hence the association of disease with ponds, lakes, dams, and irrigation systems. Children aged 5 to 15 years are at greatest risk, largely due to frequent recreational exposure in freshwater bodies infested by intermediate host snails.

PATHOPHYSIOLOGY

Transmission to children is via cutaneous invasion by tiny cercariae released into water from *Bulinus* (*S haematobium*), *Biomphalaria* (*S mansoni*), or *Oncomelania* (*S japonicum*) snails. Following penetration, parasites travel hematogenously to the intrahepatic portal system, where adults mature and mate over 1 to 3 months. *S haematobium* organisms then migrate to venous channels of the bladder, and intestinal species make their way to the lower mesenteric veins. Adult worms are 1- to 2-cm long and remain intravascular for the duration of their multiyear life span. Female flukes produce up to several hundred eggs daily, which are responsible for the most severe pathology. Eggs breach vessel walls and adjacent tissue to enter

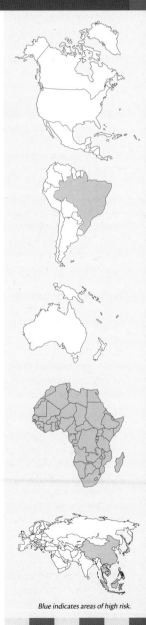

Blue indicates areas of high risk.

bladder or intestinal lumens. Eggs then pass with urine (*S haematobium*) or stool (*S mansoni, S japonicum*), hatch in water to release mobile miracidia, and lead to snail infection—completing the life cycle. Other eggs, usually in clusters, stimulate a vigorous tissue granulomatous reaction and inflammatory response. Epithelioid and giant cells, eosinophils, and lymphocytes form concentric lesions around eggs, measuring up to several centimeters in diameter. In the urinary system, these grow on bladder mucosa, at ureteropelvic junctions, or inside ureters and contribute to fibrosis and calcification. Obstructive uropathy, hydronephrosis and, in severe cases, renal failure result. Bladder cancer may also occur in advanced cases. Many light intestinal infections are asymptomatic. Heavier worm loads lead to colonic pseudopolyposis, portal hypertension, and hepatosplenomegaly. Hepatocellular function is remarkably well preserved initially but, in late stages, hepatic cirrhosis and cor pulmonale result. Other organs, including the brain, spinal cord, lung, heart, and bone, are involved rarely. Some degree of acquired immunity seems to develop among those repeatedly infected.

CLINICAL PRESENTATION

Acute symptoms are most intense in immunologically naive children suffering heavy parasitic loads. Cercarial dermatitis is a pruritic, maculopapular, self-limiting rash appearing at the site of cercariae skin entry 1 to 2 days after penetration. Acute schistosomiasis coincides with fluke maturation in the weeks and months following infection and is characterized by a serum sickness-like syndrome of fever, anorexia, abdominal pain, cough, myalgias, lymphadenopathy, and hepatomegaly. A particularly serious form of acute disease was once reported in southern Japan's Katayama Valley.

Chronic symptoms manifest months to years after exposure and stem from immune reactions against eggs lodged in tissue with inflammation, granuloma formation, and scarring. Urinary schistosomiasis presents with terminal hematuria, dysuria, and symptoms of ureteral obstruction. Intestinal and hepatosplenic schistosomiasis may be asymptomatic or lead to nonspecific weakness and weight loss. In heavy infections, abdominal cramps, dysentery, and hepatosplenomegaly are common. Later, esophageal varices from portal hypertension and, ultimately, liver failure develop.

Neuroschistosomiasis, presenting with seizures, encephalitis, or myelitis, is caused by worm migration to the central nervous system. Flukes trekking to other atypical organs cause localized pulmonary, cardiac, or bony symptoms.

Repeated infections exert a collective toll on children's growth and development, with gradual weakening and fatigue, anemia, nutritional deficiencies, stunting, and cognitive impairment.

DIAGNOSIS

Chronic urinary and gastrointestinal infection are confirmed by microscopic identification of eggs in urine or stool. Diagnosis is often facilitated by urine sedimentation or filtration, or by stool concentration techniques. Examination of rectal biopsy specimens may also demonstrate eggs. Peripheral eosinophilia is a regular finding. Serologic testing is available. Acute infection is chiefly a clinical diagnosis because eggs are not yet excreted and antibody titers not yet elevated.

TREATMENT AND PREVENTION

Praziquantel is the treatment of choice for all forms of schistosomiasis and generally results in high cure and egg reduction rates. Those not fully cured often still benefit from considerable reduction in worm burden. Early detection and treatment can prevent progression to chronic disease manifestations, although some late-stage sequelae (eg, renal failure) are irreversible.

Preventing or limiting schistosomiasis is accomplished by avoiding freshwater contact in endemic areas (chlorinated pools and ocean water are safe), reducing persistent water contamination by promoting improved hygienic practices, periodic mass chemotherapy, and snail control by molluscacide.

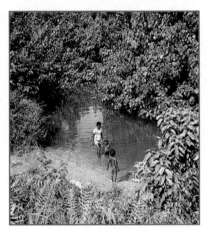

IMAGE 1

A refreshing swim on a hot day may seem appealing to children but carries the risk of acquiring schistosomiasis in endemic areas. Occupational exposure, for example among fisherman and irrigation workers, also puts select older populations in peril. Schistosomiasis is the most important helminth infection in terms of human pathology. Malaria is arguably the only tropical parasitic disease that is more devastating. *Courtesy: Jose Fierro.*

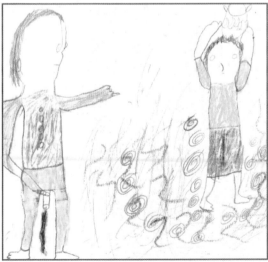

IMAGE 2

A child in western Cote d'Ivoire shares an understanding of the community's affliction in a simple and poignant manner. The graphic representation of snails, worms, rash, and hematuria are unmistakable. *Courtesy: Juerg Utzinger.*

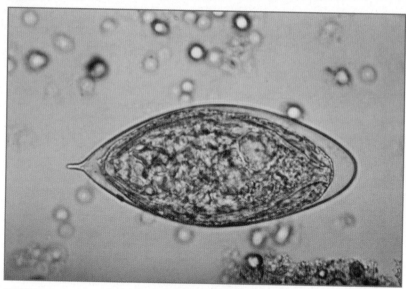

IMAGE 3

A magnified view of a *Schistosoma haematobium* egg. The terminal spine is a distinguishing feature of this species. Ova are transmitted by human urine or stool into freshwater bodies, where they hatch and release miracidia. Snails host further development of the parasite. *Courtesy: Centers for Disease Control and Prevention.*

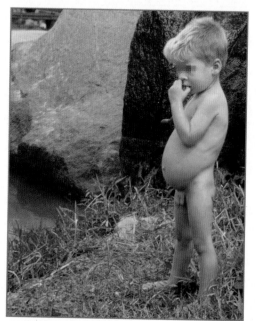

IMAGE 4

A Puerto Rican boy with a swollen abdomen due to Bilharzia. The common name for schistosomiasis is tribute to Theodor Bilharz, who first reported the disease in the mid-1800s. Schistosomiasis, however, has been around much longer than that: Schistosoma ova were identified in ancient Egyptian and Chinese mummies. *Courtesy: Centers for Disease Control and Prevention.*

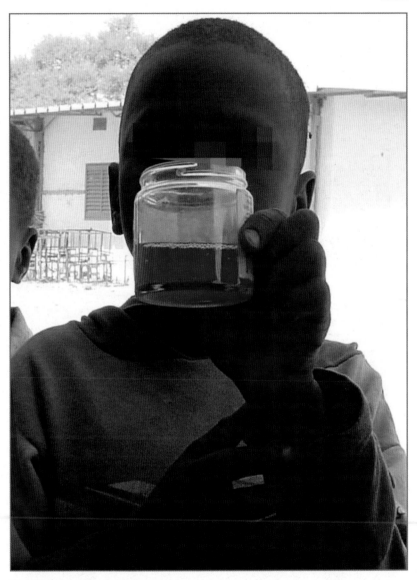

IMAGE 5

A school child from Niger suffers gross hematuria from urinary schistosomiasis. *Schistosoma haematobium* is most prevalent in Africa and the Middle East. *Schistosoma mansoni* is also found in Africa and is the only species observed in Latin America and the Caribbean. *Schistosoma japonicum* is restricted to the Pacific region (including China and the Philippines), *Schistosoma intercalatum* occurs in 10 countries in the rainforest belt of Africa, and *Schistosoma mekongi* is found in limited areas of Laos and Cambodia.
Courtesy: Juerg Utzinger.

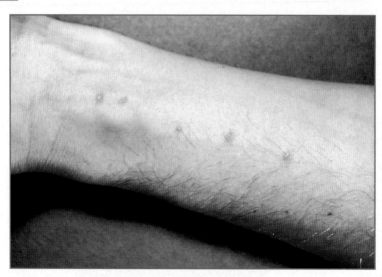

IMAGE 6

Swimmer's, or *clam digger's, itch* is a papular rash that follows cutaneous penetration of free-swimming cercaria. Dermatitis is more common in travelers compared with residents of endemic areas. *Courtesy: Centers for Disease Control and Prevention.*

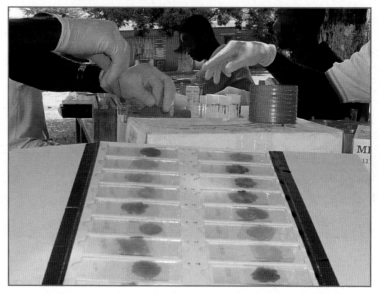

IMAGE 7

Field diagnosis of intestinal schistosomiasis is commonly made by stool examination. Direct smears have low sensitivity. Preparation of Kato-Katz thick smears is a concentration technique used to improve the diagnostic yield. *Courtesy: Juerg Utzinger.*

Scurvy

BACKGROUND

Outbreaks of scurvy, a relatively rare disease of Vitamin C (also known as ascorbic acid) deficiency have been primarily associated over the past 3 decades with internally displaced and refugee populations that have been denied food access because of war or conflict. These groups were removed from their normal source of vitamin C (eg, camel's milk, tomatoes, sweet potatoes) or relied on emergency food rations that may have been inadequately fortified with vitamin C and other micronutrients. Prevalence rates of scurvy in refugee camps in the 1990s ranged from 10% to 40% and were among the highest recorded for the 20th century. Risk of scurvy in displaced populations depends on length of time in camp (clinical scurvy often occurs 3–4 months after arrival) and is higher in the elderly and in women of reproductive age, especially if pregnant.

PATHOPHYSIOLOGY

Humans cannot synthesize ascorbic acid and remain dependent on intestinal absorption for this essential nutrient. In the absence of adequate intake, body stores of vitamin C will be lost within 2 to 3 months. Severe deficiency leads to the breakdown of intercellular cement substances and defective growth of collagen, osteoid, and dentine. Depletion of pericapillary collagen results in capillary hemorrhages. Larger cerebral, pericardial, or myocardial bleeds can be fatal in untreated children. Vitamin C also plays an important role in immune system function, and scurvy is associated with an increased risk of bacterial and mycobacterial infections.

CLINICAL PRESENTATION

Early signs are fatigue and myalgias. Weakness follows, and evolves into an irritable lethargy. Discomfort worsens with movement. Frank bone pain from subperiosteal hemorrhage, loosening of secondary teeth, and intradermal and gingival hemorrhage may occur as the disease progresses. Other symptoms include anorexia, low-grade fever, mild diarrhea, and hematochezia. Severe and prolonged scurvy results in

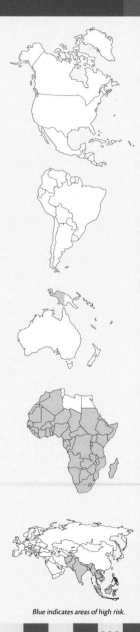

Blue indicates areas of high risk.

skeletal muscle degeneration, cardiac hypertrophy, adrenal hypertrophy, and diminished bone marrow function. Anemia is common from a combination of blood loss, folate deficiency, and decreased iron absorption. Dermatologic manifestations include petechiae, ecchymoses, follicular hyperkeratosis, and "corkscrew" hairs. Wound healing is delayed. Ocular manifestations include conjunctival and intraocular hemorrhages.

In contrast to adults, bone disease is a frequent manifestation of scurvy in children and can be debilitating. Infants may present with lassitude, irritability, and frog-legged or pithed-frog position of pseudoparalysis with external rotation of the lower extremities. Older children present with bone pain, limping, leg swelling, occult fracture (especially around the growth plates), or inability to walk. Subluxation of the sternum at the costochondral junctions is very common in infants and may produce palpable swellings known as *scorbutic beads,* resembling the rachitic rosary of rickets. The sternum in children with scurvy is typically depressed.

DIAGNOSIS

Diagnosis of scurvy is largely made on clinical grounds. The constellation of bone and gingival disease, hyperkeratosis, and petechiae or purpura is highly suggestive in a child with a history of dietary inadequacy of vitamin C.

In most tropical settings, sophisticated laboratory evaluation is not available or necessary. If performed, serum ascorbate levels are specific but not sensitive. Measures of urinary excretion of ascorbic acid after parenteral ascorbic acid challenge is a more sensitive sign of deficiency. Patients with normal vitamin C levels will excrete greater than 80% of an intravenous challenge. Radiologic findings of bone demineralization in infantile scurvy are typical. Classic ground glass osteopenia appears as a line of increased density surrounding the epiphysis, and Pelkan spurs at the periphery of the zone of calcification result from healing metaphyseal fractures. With periosteal bleeding, extensive new bone is seen along the shafts of the long bones.

TREATMENT AND PREVENTION

Concomitant nutritional deficiencies of vitamins A and B_6, iron, and folate must be considered along with other complications of acute and chronic malnutrition. In displaced populations, scurvy can be avoided by the distribution of fresh foods, fortification of relief food, supplementation of a multivitamin supplying micronutrients, and promotion of kitchen gardens (especially in long-term camps). The definitive treatment is administering ascorbic acid. Response is often dramatic. Bleeding, irritability, and bone pain can resolve within 12 to 48 hours.

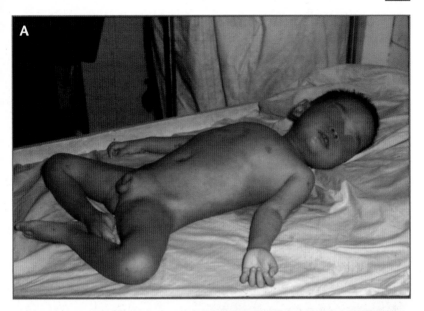

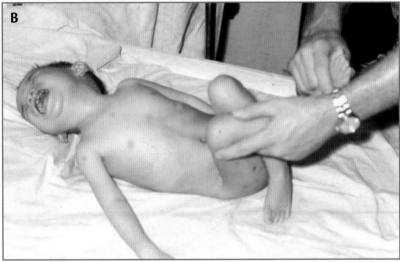

IMAGE 1A, 1B

A young boy with scurvy demonstrates lethargy, irritability, pithed-frog position of the lower extremities, and scattered small ecchymoses and petechiae. Bony pain worsened dramatically with movement of extremities. The child became symptom-free within 12 hours of parenteral Vitamin C. *Courtesy: Frederick M. Burkle Jr.*

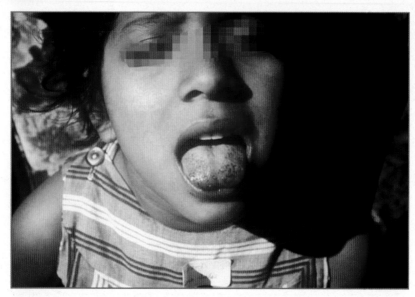

IMAGE 2

Scorbutic tongue is characterized by glossitis, erythema, and submucosal hemorrhages.
Courtesy: Centers for Disease Control and Prevention.

Snakebite

BACKGROUND

Snakebites are a major cause of morbidity and mortality in tropical regions although they receive relatively limited attention. Five million snakebites are estimated to occur worldwide each year, resulting in roughly 2.5 million envenomations, approximately 100,000 deaths, and 150,000 nonfatal but serious sequellae. In Southeast Asia and Africa, snake envenomation accounts for approximately 50,000 deaths annually, many of which are not reported to formal health systems. Fifteen percent of all snakes are venomous, and they cause more human fatalities than all other venomous and poisonous animals combined.

In developing countries, snakebites are a familiar occupational hazard, particularly among agricultural workers, fishermen, and hunters. Behavioral patterns put school-aged children and males at greater risk. In all age groups, most bites occur on the extremities, usually the legs and feet. Medically important venomous snakes include elapids (eg, cobras, mambas, coral snakes, and kraits), true vipers (eg, Old World vipers, adders), and pit vipers (eg, New World vipers, copperheads, rattlesnakes, and water moccasins).

PATHOPHYSIOLOGY

Snakes inject venom, a form of toxic and digestive saliva, through modified glands and tubular fangs. The clinical signs and symptoms of envenomations result from pathogenic proteins, including neurotoxins, cardiotoxins, hemotoxins, and myotoxins.

CLINICAL PRESENTATION

Signs and symptoms of snake envenomation vary considerably between individual patients with regard to reaction types, timing of onset, and course of illness. Local tissue and muscle damage ranges from edema, bruising, and blistering to severe necrosis. Though rare, certain snakes (namely spitting cobras and the ringhals) propel venom into the eyes of their victim causing pain and irritation, a condition known as *cobra spit ophthalmia*. In severe cases, conjunctivitis and corneal damage lead to permanent visual impairment.

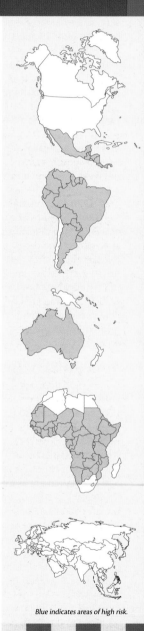

Blue indicates areas of high risk.

The most common systemic reaction to snakebite is fear, which itself can cause nausea, tachycardia, clammy skin, and syncope. Nonspecific signs of envenomation include headache, vomiting, and abdominal pain. Specific effects of toxic snakebites are determined by the components of injected venom. Neurotoxins and hemotoxins are the most common and life-threatening. Neurotoxins trigger a descending paralysis, progressing from ophthalmoplegia and ptosis to swallowing difficulties, slurred speech, weakness, respiratory paralysis, and cardiac arrest. Total flaccid paralysis and locked-in syndrome may occur. Hemotoxins are characterized by anti-hemostatic effects and can set off spontaneous bleeding, hypotension, shock, and death. Cardiotoxins damage myocardial tissue and contribute to shock. Myotoxins lead to muscle pain, rhabdomyolysis, and acute renal failure. Children are especially vulnerable to severe systemic complications given their smaller size and limited communication capacity.

DIAGNOSIS

Up to one-half of potentially toxic snakebites do not result in envenomation (so-called dry bites). The confirmation of envenomation therefore depends on close clinical monitoring. A rapid, detailed history should be taken as the child's airway, breathing, and circulation are assessed. Identifying the snake type through descriptive means can be useful for predicting likelihood of disease severity. The skin around the bite should be examined for fang or tooth marks, scratches, edema, and bruising. Baseline and serial circumference measurements above and below the site are useful to monitor swelling and guide therapy. In settings where laboratory studies are available, baseline evaluation often includes a complete blood count, coagulation profile, fibrin degradation products, electrolytes, blood urea nitrogen, serum creatinine, and urinalysis. A simple bedside clotting time can be measured by placing blood in a clean, dry glass tube; if the blood does not clot after sitting undisturbed for 20 minutes, the test is abnormal.

TREATMENT AND PREVENTION

In remote areas, immediate first aid should include immobilization of the bitten limb to inhibit potentially destructive venom from reaching the systemic circulation. Transport to a medical facility is recommended because optimal management of snakebite victims may require aggressive supportive care and sometimes the administration of antivenin.

A number of "therapeutic" practices that were popular in the past are now known to be useless or even harmful to snakebite victims. Incision, excision, placing a tourniquet, electric shock, chemical injection, local freezing, suctioning, and applying a "snake-stone" (which purports to draw venom from the wound) should *not* be performed. Pressure immobilization, however, can be lifesaving by lessening or delaying toxin effect. The technique involves careful bandaging of the affected limb, beginning at the fingers or toes and working proximally, similar to the process of wrapping a sprained ankle. Sufficient pressure should obstruct lymphatics without compromising blood flow. To avoid ischemia, the bandage should be loosened at once if peripheral pulses are diminished, pain increases, or the limb becomes discolored.

Antivenins are antibodies to snake venom epitopes that are obtained from hyperimmunized animal sources (eg, horses and sheep) and represent an additional invaluable treatment adjunct. In cases of elapid snakebite, immediate therapy with appropriate antivenin is warranted in virtually all cases because associated paralysis can be prevented but not reversed. In the event of cytotoxic or hemotoxic envenomation, mild local swelling alone may not warrant undertaking the risk of allergic complications that can be seen with antivenin, but benefits outweigh risks in severe cases. Its use should be considered in the presence of spontaneous systemic bleeding, shock, paralysis, dark or bloody urine, swelling involving more than half the bitten limb, or envenomation to areas vulnerable to necrosis such as the distal extremities.

Fluid management, renal dialysis, and assisted ventilation may be required in some children. Tetanus prophylaxis should be administered. Bacterial superinfection is not uncommon. Following severe snake envenomation, surgical debridement and fasciotomy is at times necessary to manage compartment syndrome but should not precede the resolution of clotting disorders.

Preventing snake envenomation is preferable to treating it. The risk of sustaining snakebites can be reduced significantly by avoiding snake habitats when possible, wearing protective footwear and clothing, and sleeping off the ground and under a mosquito net.

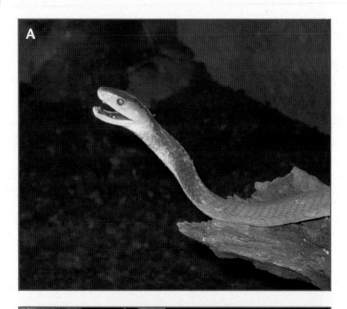

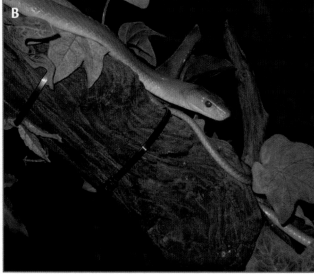

IMAGE 1A, 1B

The black and green mambas (*Dendroaspis polylepis* and *Dendroaspis viridis,* respectively) inject venom with high levels of neurotoxin and are therefore considered among Africa's most dangerous snakes. Note that the black mamba is actually metallic in color rather than black. *Courtesy: B. Ryan Phelps.*

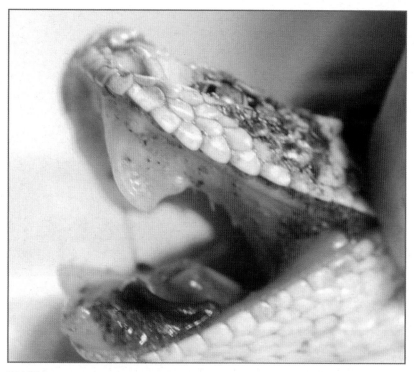

IMAGE 2

The tubular, fleshy fangs of pit vipers are hinged and hollow. They retract against the roof of the mouth when not in use. Pit vipers are so named for the small pit located between their eyes and nostrils that detects heat and enables nighttime hunting. *Courtesy: Norberto Sotelo Cruz.*

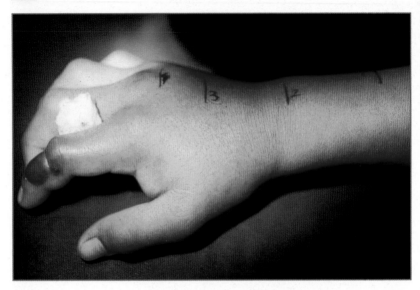

IMAGE 3

Localized swelling and bruising over a digit is evident following envenomation. The monitoring of this patient, who received antivenin to protect the finger, included measuring and marking the swelling at regular intervals to determine whether additional antivenin would be required. Unfortunately, modern antivenins are often unavailable in areas of the world with the highest burden of disease from venomous snakebites, and many health centers rely on supportive care alone or older generations of antivenin. *Courtesy: Norberto Sotelo Cruz.*

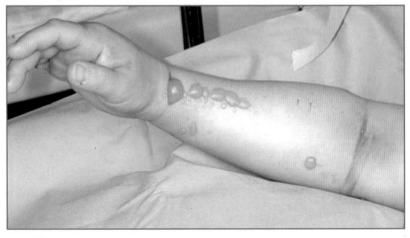

IMAGE 4

A pit viper bite to the hand was complicated by rapid progression of tenderness and blistering along the lymphatic chain and bruising in the antecubital fossa. *Courtesy: Tim Strubel.*

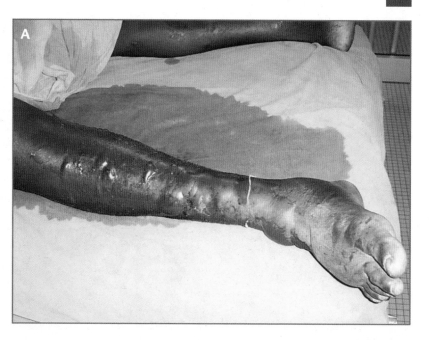

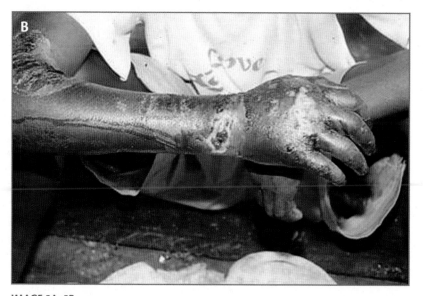

IMAGE 5A, 5B

Advanced extremity envenomation sequellae are seen in the days following puff adder (Image 5A) and Gaboon viper (Image 5B) bites. Progressive blistering and necrosis are evident.
Courtesy: Jean-Philippe Chippaux (Image 5A) and Cellou Balde (Image 5B).

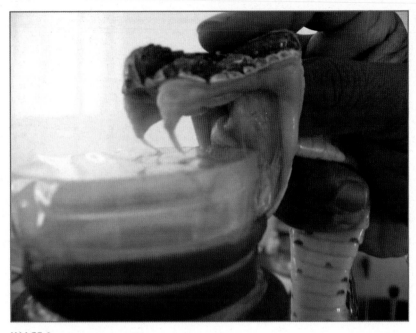

IMAGE 6

A Russell viper (*Vipera russelii*) is milked for venom at a Sri Lankan laboratory to produce antivenin. *Courtesy: Rais Vohra.*

Tetanus

COMMON NAME

Lockjaw

BACKGROUND

Tetanus is caused by the gram-positive bacillus *Clostridium tetani*. The organism is an obligate anaerobe yet is ubiquitous in the environment in the form of remarkably resilient spores. Soil and feces (animal and human) are well-established reservoirs. Approximately 1 million cases occur annually, nearly half in newborns in whom mortality rates are particularly high—near 90%. Populations with low rates of immunization coverage are at greatest risk.

PATHOPHYSIOLOGY

C tetani spores exhibit resistance to extreme weather conditions and disinfectants. They can survive virtually forever in an inactive state but require anaerobic conditions for germination. Deep, necrotic soft tissue wounds constitute an ideal medium for bacterium vegetation and replication. Invasive bacilli elaborate a potent neurotoxin, tetanospasmin, which irreversibly blocks release of inhibitory neurotransmitters (γ-aminobutyric acid and glycine) at myoneural junctions. Unrepressed muscular excitation results. Toxin can migrate from the site of contamination to the spinal cord and brain in a matter of days and cause autonomic instability and generalized disease. Heavily contaminated wounds are associated with shorter incubations, more severe illness, and a worse prognosis.

CLINICAL PRESENTATION

Tetanus follows infection of a dirty wound or, in the case of newborns, a contaminated umbilical cord. No source is identified in up to one-third of children. *C tetani* does not itself elicit a robust host inflammatory response or tissue damage. After an incubation period ranging from several days to weeks, disease manifests as one of the following clinical syndromes.

Generalized Tetanus

Patients present with trismus, or lockjaw, resulting from masseter muscle rigidity. Muscular spasms in the

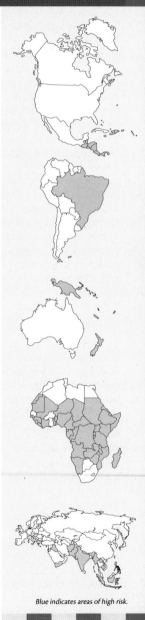

Blue indicates areas of high risk.

head and neck give way to sustained contraction of facial muscles and characteristic risus sardonicus (a fixed appearance of scornful laughter). Symptoms progress to widespread body rigidity and painful spasms in response to physical, visual, auditory, and aural stimuli. Opisthotonic posturing is typical. Involvement of laryngeal muscles and the diaphragm may cause upper airway obstruction or respiratory failure. Deep tendon reflexes are hyperactive, and spasms may be so strong as to rip tendons or break bones. Signs of autonomic dysfunction include blood pressure and heart rate fluctuations, profuse sweating, and fever. Consciousness is maintained. Generalized tetanus develops over 1 to 7 days, remains severe for a week or two and, in survivors, resolves over the next month. Mortality rates are up to 60%. Disease does not confer immunity, and recurrences are possible in the absence of active immunization.

Localized Tetanus

Localized tetanus presents as mild persistent rigidity and pain localized to muscles close to the site of spore inoculation. Symptoms can persist for months and resolve spontaneously but, without treatment, disease may also generalize.

Cephalic Tetanus

This is a rare form of tetanus, secondary to head-penetrating trauma or otitis media, causing cranial nerve palsies. Generalization may occur.

Neonatal Tetanus

Infection is a consequence of poor umbilical hygiene and lack of maternal immunization. Irritability and poor feeding usually manifest by a week of age and herald intense muscular spasms, rigidity, and apnea. Sensory stimulation worsens symptoms. The baby will be unable to eat and, many times, will lose the ability to breathe spontaneously. Autonomic disturbances are common.

DIAGNOSIS

Tetanus is a clinical diagnosis. Distinguishing features in older children are sustained facial muscle contraction and opisthotonus. Newborns are rigid and unable to interact appropriately. As a rule, laboratory investigations are not helpful, although a positive *C tetani* wound culture can contribute supportive evidence of infection. Cerebrospinal fluid is normal except for increased opening pressure, especially during spasms.

TREATMENT AND PREVENTION

Wounds should be cleaned and debrided. Passive and active immunization is indicated if tetanus is suspected and must be administered as soon as possible. Intramuscular tetanus immune globulin (TIG) provides passive immunity and may decrease both disease course and severity. A single dose is delivered preferably at 2 sites near the wound. Where TIG is unavailable, equine tetanus antitoxin may be used after sensitivity testing and desensitization. Active immunization is achieved with tetanus toxoid given as DTP, Tdap, or Td vaccine. Antibiotics have no effect on tetanospasmin but are required to eradicate bacilli. Metronidazole or penicillin is the agent of choice. Patients with localized or cephalic tetanus should be treated immediately to decrease the likelihood of disease progression.

Supportive treatment can be lifesaving in patients with generalized tetanus. Minimizing external stimulation is critical. Patients are frequently cared for in dark, quiet, isolated rooms. Mainstays of symptomatic therapy for muscle spasms and rigidity are benzodiazepines, which indirectly antagonize the effects of tetanospasmin. Narcotics, barbiturates, paralytics, and muscle relaxants are sometimes also used. Ventilatory and nutritional support (eg, nasogastric tube feeding) are often required.

Management of neonatal tetanus is extremely challenging even in countries that benefit from sophisticated medical services, hence its dramatic fatality rate in resource-limited settings. Approach to care is similar to the treatment of older patients with generalized disease: sensory tranquility, TIG, fluid and nutritional support, and mechanical ventilation if needed. Patients will require active tetanus immunization as well. Treatment of spasms must be weighed against monitoring abilities so that iatrogenic respiratory cessation does not occur.

Preventing disease altogether is by far the most important strategy for decreasing tetanus-associated morbidity and mortality. Concentrated effort should support national childhood immunization programs. Pregnancy is not a contraindication to tetanus vaccination. On the contrary, immunization status during pregnancy should be assessed and vaccine administered to unimmunized women.

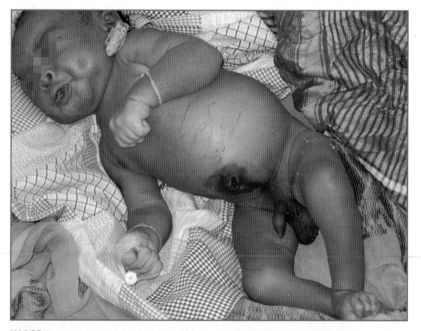

IMAGE 1

Sustained muscle contraction of the face and body is apparent in this 7-day-old with neonatal tetanus. Gentian violet antiseptic coats the infected umbilicus. Traditional newborn care practices in some parts of the world may in fact contribute to risk of disease by soiling the umbilical cord with a dirty blade, grass, or manure. The condition is painful and usually fatal in infants and is heartbreaking to parents and caregivers who understand that the illness is completely preventable.

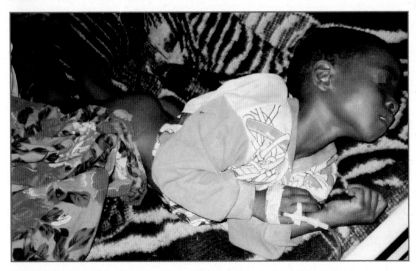

IMAGE 2

A young boy with opisthotonos in sub-Saharan Africa. Convex spasm of the spine may be accompanied by flexion and adduction of arms, clenching of fists, and extension of lower extremities.

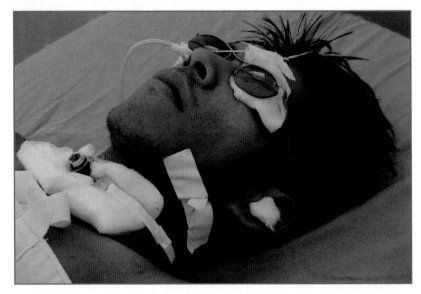

IMAGE 3

Painful tetanic spasms are triggered by external stimuli including light and sound. Eye shades and ear plugs helped to decrease provocation in this adolescent suffering from generalized tetanus in rural Peru. Nasogastric feedings were delivered, and a tracheotomy was placed due to concerns for respiratory compromise. *Courtesy: Michael Dinerman.*

Tinea

COMMON NAMES

Athlete's foot, Jock itch, Ringworm, Serpigo

BACKGROUND

Tinea denotes dermatophytosis, a fungal infection of the skin, hair, or nails. By convention, further classification is dictated by lesion location (eg, tinea barbae [beard], capitis [scalp and hair shaft], corporis [body], cruris [groin], manus [palmar hand], pedis [foot], and unguium [nail bed]). Tinea is extremely common worldwide, especially in the warm humidity of the tropics. *Microsporum, Trichophyton,* and *Epidermophyton* are frequently implicated genera. Dermatophytes are acquired through person-to-person contact, via fomites, or from infected animals or soil.

Tinea versicolor is now referred to as *pityriasis,* is caused by *Malassezia furfur*, and is characterized by circumscribed, pigmented scales on the upper body.

PATHOPHYSIOLOGY

Only keratinized surfaces are affected; mucosa is spared. A predilection for moist or macerated areas occurs, hence involvement of areas such as the groin or spaces between the toes. Host defense mechanisms play an important role in helping to limit fungal invasion to superficial cutaneous tissue.

CLINICAL PRESENTATION

Affected sites have distinct symptomatology. Pruritis is a common finding in most forms of the disease.

Tinea capitis presents in various ways. Areas of alopecia with scaling similar to dandruff may occur. Lesions often coalesce into thick, white, rough plaques with a powdery appearance. Infection of hair shafts may cause hair to break off close to the base, leaving patches of black dot studs on the scalp. Tinea capitis can also be erythematous, and nuchal lymphadenopathy is frequently present. Occasionally, a severe inflammatory response develops and takes the form of a large boggy mass, a kerion, which can be mistaken for cellulitis or a subcutaneous abscess. Kerions can lead to permanent scarring and hair loss.

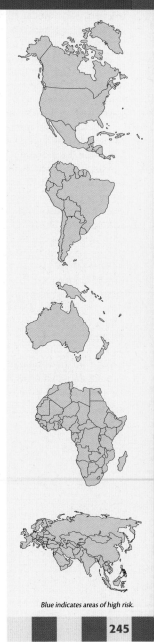

Blue indicates areas of high risk.

Tinea corporis manifests initially as a red, scaly plaque that then spreads centrifugally with central clearing, giving rise to an annular appearance. The advancing edge remains erythematous with papules or small pustules.

Tinea cruris presents with sharply demarcated, erythematous plaques that are typically symmetrical, involving the intertriginous regions of the groin, buttocks, thighs, and scrotum.

Tinea unguium is distinguished by thickened, flaking nails, usually with a yellowish discoloration.

Note that fungal pathogens such as tinea occasionally provoke a hypersensitivity id reaction characterized by a vesicular or pustular dermatitis of the extremities, trunk, or face (most common with tinea capitis or pedis).

DIAGNOSIS

Classic lesions require no special evaluation, and diagnosis can be made on clinical grounds alone. The fungi of tinea capitis may fluoresce with Wood light examination. Wet mounts of skin scrapings can be examined microscopically; hyphae will be visualized with addition of potassium hydroxide. When necessary, for instance with resistant cases, definitive dermatophyte identification can be obtained by culture.

TREATMENT AND PREVENTION

Tinea corporis, cruris, and pedis generally respond to prolonged courses (2–6 weeks) of topical antifungals such as clotrimazole or ketoconazole. Resistant cases may necessitate oral therapy. Hair and nail infections are impervious to topical agents and should be treated with oral medications for a month or more, usually griseofulvin (for capitis), terbinafine (for unguium), or an oral azole (for unguium). Kerions are also managed with griseofulvin; steroids may be a useful adjunct but antibiotics are required only in the presence of secondary bacterial infection. Pityriasis is treated with topical selenium sulfide lotion or shampoo, topical antifungals, or short courses of oral antifungals.

Good hygiene is principal to tinea prevention. Sharing clothing, towels, etc, with others who are affected is to be avoided. Potential animal sources should be identified and treated. Keeping at-risk body areas dry with an absorbent powder is beneficial (especially the groin and feet). Unfortunately, recurrence rates are high.

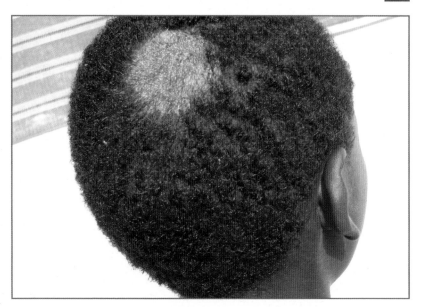

IMAGE 1

Tinea capitis in a young boy in Ethiopia. Treatment was with griseofulvin for 4 to 6 weeks. Griseofulvin bioavailability may be increased when ingested immediately following a high-fat meal.

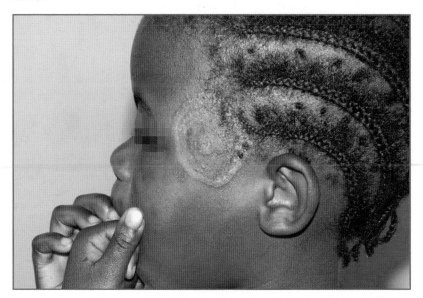

IMAGE 2

A Kenyan girl with tinea corporis. *Courtesy: Geoffrey Garst.*

Toxocariasis

COMMON NAMES

Ocular larva migrans, Visceral larva migrans

BACKGROUND

Toxocariasis is a zoonosis acquired from common roundworms of canines and felines, particularly *Toxocara canis* and *Toxocara cati*. Human infection follows accidental ingestion of embryonate eggs in soil, and disease is most common in children aged 1 to 4 years with a history of pica and puppy exposure. Older children playing in sandboxes and other areas potentially contaminated by animal feces are also at risk. Distribution is worldwide.

PATHOPHYSIOLOGY

Female dogs and cats constitute an important *Toxocara* reservoir. Infection is reactivated during pregnancy, and organisms are subsequently transmitted to puppies and kittens through the placenta and nursed milk. Most eggs passed into the environment are from infant puppies and their lactating mothers. Eggs become infective after approximately 3 weeks in soil and remain viable for months.

Following ingestion of eggs by children, larvae hatch, penetrate the gastrointestinal mucosa, and are swept up by the portal and then systemic circulations. Prolonged larval migration usually ends in the eye, liver, lung, heart, muscle, or brain. Clinical manifestations stem from damage induced by larvae and host reactions including localized eosinophilic granulomatosis. Size of the ingested larval load and degree of host reactivity are primary factors in symptom severity. Humans do not excrete *Toxocara* eggs.

CLINICAL MANIFESTATIONS

Most children with light infections are asymptomatic. Three main clinical syndromes exist.

Visceral Larva Migrans (VLM)

Children with VLM have fever, hepatomegaly, leukocytosis, and hypergammaglobulinemia. Splenomegaly, lymphadenopathy, and myocarditis are also possible. A clinical syndrome similar to asthma can develop with

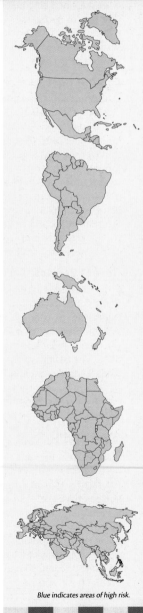

Blue indicates areas of high risk.

cough, bronchospasm, patchy alveolar infiltrates, and hypereosinophilia. Less commonly, patients present with cutaneous signs (including hemorrhagic rash, urticaria, or nodules) or neurologic complications (such as focal or generalized seizures, behavioral disorders, or subtle neurologic deficits).

Ocular Larva Migrans (OLM)

Ocular larva migrans affects slightly older children, usually 5 to 10 years of age, who present with unilateral visual impairment or strabismus. Retina invasion by the parasite leads to granuloma formation, typically in the periphery or posterior pole, and leads to retinal traction and potential detachment and blindness. Ocular larva migrans can also result in leukocoria, endophthalmitis, papillitis, uveitis, and secondary glaucoma. Systemic manifestations are rare.

Covert Toxocariasis

Covert disease is a frequently undiagnosed condition described by serologic evidence of toxocariasis in patients with mild, nonspecific, or no symptoms. Children may present with pulmonary disease including wheezing, acute bronchitis, and pneumonitis; dermatologic findings such as chronic urticaria or eczema; chronic abdominal pain; lymphadenopathy; myositis; or arthralgias.

DIAGNOSIS

Visceral larva migrans should be suspected in children with epidemiological risk factors, typical symptoms, marked leukocytosis, and eosinophilia. Serology is helpful. Definitive diagnosis is by histologic examination of involved tissue but is rarely indicated.

The diagnosis of OLM is also based on clinical manifestations in at-risk children. A positive serum enzyme-linked immunosorbent assay for *Toxocara* IgG is supportive, although this assay is less sensitive for the diagnosis of OLM than for other forms of toxocariasis. Aqueous or vitreous fluid examination can be useful in select cases because antibody titers within this space are typically higher compared with serum. Eosinophilia is often absent.

Covert toxocariasis is diagnosed in individuals with nonspecific symptoms accompanied by elevated IgE titers, eosinophilia, and positive *Toxocara* serology.

Imaging techniques can be used to detect and localize granulomatous lesions due to *Toxocara* larvae. Multiple hypoechoic liver lesions may be demonstrated by abdominal ultrasound. On computed tomography, these appear as low-density infiltrates. Ocular ultrasound may show a highly reflective peripheral mass, vitreous bands or membranes, or traction retinal detachment.

TREATMENT AND PREVENTION

Management of patients with mild VLM and covert disease is controversial. Many infections are self-limited and may not require specific therapy. More severe disease is treated with albendazole or mebendazole in conjunction with steroids, bronchodilators, and antihistamines. Topical or systemic steroids are indicated for OLM; antiparasitics have not consistently been shown to be of significant additional benefit. Laser photocoagulation can help destroy larvae in the eye, and surgery may be required to manage ocular complications.

Preventive measures include regular deworming of dogs and cats (especially puppies and kittens), stopping pica behaviors, maintenance of clean child play areas, and ensuring good handwashing after children spend time outside in regions of high endemicity.

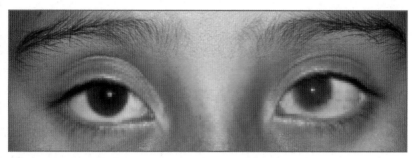

IMAGE 1

Ocular toxocariasis in an 8-year-old boy who suffered from progressive loss of visual acuity in his left eye for 10 months followed by strabismus. He lived with a dog and cat and had a history of geophagia. Hypereosinophilia was present, and serum IgE was elevated 20-fold. Convalescent ELISA titers were positive. Note the presence of a cyclitic membrane covering the left pupil. Posterior uveitis led to glaucoma of the same eye. *Courtesy: Ciro Maguiña.*

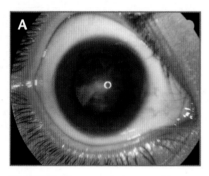
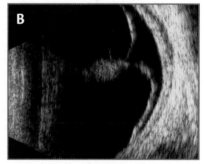

IMAGE 2A, 2B

An 11-year-old child with ocular toxocariasis. Progressive unilateral vision loss of 3 years' duration was accompanied by headache and strabismus. Funduscopic examination revealed a peripheral granuloma with fibrous tracts projecting from the papillae. Leukocoria is evident (Image 2A). Ocular ultrasound demonstrates the same granuloma and retinal detachment (Image 2B). Convalescent *Toxocara canis* titers were positive and serum IgE was markedly elevated. *Courtesy: Luis Tobaru and Isaias Rolando (Image 2A); Mario de la Torre (Image 2B).*

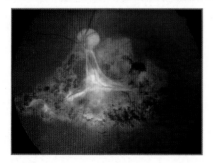

IMAGE 3

Funduscopy in an adolescent female who complained of visual acuity reduction and strabismus. Geophagia was denied but a dog and cat lived in the household. A granuloma is visible at the posterior pole with fibrotic tracts and a neovascular choroid membrane. Serology was positive. *Courtesy: Luis Tobaru and Isaias Rolando.*

Toxoplasmosis

BACKGROUND

Toxoplasma gondii is a highly adaptable intracellular parasite with a broad worldwide distribution. Up to a third of the human population has been infected. Prevalence rates are highest in warm and humid climates, which favor survival of oocytes. Cows, sheep, pigs, and other warm-blooded vertebrates are important reservoirs of disease, but only felines host the organism's sexual stage of development. Five percent of cattle and 25% of pigs in the United States are thought to harbor *T gondii*, and the burden is likely much higher in many less developed parts of the world. Human infection results following exposure to infected cat feces, consumption of raw meat, or vertical transmission through the placenta. Acquired infection is common and usually asymptomatic in immunocompetent individuals. Congenital infection is less common but potentially devastating.

PATHOPHYSIOLOGY

Cats acquire *T gondii* through ingestion of infected prey. The parasite undergoes sexual differentiation in feline intestines and, days to weeks later, oocytes appear in cat feces. Millions of oocytes may be produced by a single cat over a period of weeks. Oocytes are extremely resilient and can survive in moist soil or water for months. Following accidental consumption by humans, the infective form of the organism escapes from the cyst in the intestinal lumen, invades the gastrointestinal epithelium, and disseminates through the body via hematogenous and lymphatic routes. *T gondii* tissue cysts are alternatively acquired by ingestion of undercooked meat. Symptoms develop straightaway, or cysts may lie dormant to be reactivated at a later date, as occurs if host immunity is subsequently weakened.

Primary infection with toxoplasmosis during pregnancy carries the risk of fetal transmission. *T gondii* acquired in the first trimester is less likely to be transmitted (<20%) but leads to more severe fetal and neonatal disease. Miscarriage may result. Mothers infected later in pregnancy are more likely to transmit the infection to the fetus (>60%), but symptoms are comparatively mild.

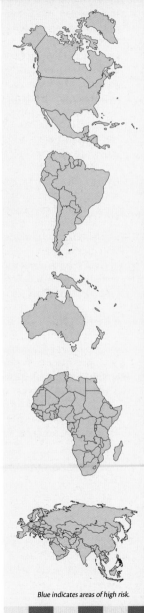

Blue indicates areas of high risk.

CLINICAL PRESENTATION

Most infections acquired in childhood are asymptomatic. Clinical signs, when they develop, most often take the form of painless cervical lymphadenopathy with or without fever. Nonspecific myalgias, nuchal rigidity, maculopapular rash, and hepatosplenomegaly occur rarely. Toxoplasmosis is considerably more serious in immunocompromised patients, in whom necrotizing encephalitis, myocarditis, and pulmonary insufficiency can be fatal. Congenitally acquired infections may be clinically obvious at birth or be subclinical for decades. Hydrocephalus, intracerebral calcifications, and chorioretinitis constitute the classic triad of congenital toxoplasmosis. Growth retardation, microcephaly, hepatosplenomegaly, thrombocytopenia, and rash may be present. Those who appear normal at birth are at risk for later development of mental deficits, chorioretinitis, and hearing loss.

DIAGNOSIS

Acute infection is generally diagnosed by serology. Microscopic examination of biopsy specimens from infected lymph nodes or the placenta can reveal organisms. Polymerase chain reaction assays for identifying *T gondii* DNA in body fluids exist but are not widely used. Where available, brain imaging is helpful for identifying hydrocephalus and intracerebral calcifications. Because symptom onset may be delayed for years, congenital toxoplasmosis should be considered in children who develop visual impairments or chorioretinitis without an obvious etiology.

TREATMENT AND PREVENTION

No treatment is required in immunocompetent children with uncomplicated, acquired toxoplasmosis. For neonates in whom congenital toxoplasmosis is confirmed, late sequelae can be mitigated by prompt and prolonged treatment with combination antibiotic therapy. Spiramycin, pyrimethamine, and sulfadiazine are the agents most commonly used. Leucovorin is given concurrently to reduce the likelihood of bone marrow suppression, which happens occasionally from pyrimethamine administration. Immunocompromised children should receive antibiotic prophylaxis to prevent infection or reactivation. Treatment of pregnant women can reduce fetal transmission, but preventing parasite acquisition during pregnancy is the most sensible approach. Steering clear of feline feces (including litter boxes and sandboxes) and avoiding the ingestion of raw meat are important educational measures in this regard.

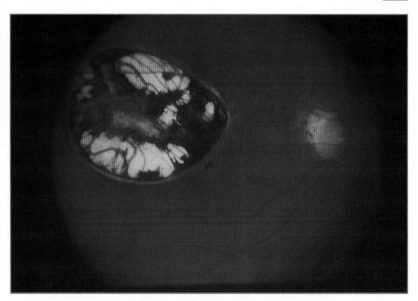

IMAGE 1

Ocular toxoplasmosis is the most common cause of chorioretinitis in immunocompetent children worldwide. White-yellow retinal infiltrates are visible. *Courtesy: Duke Duncan.*

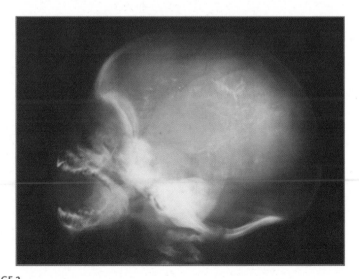

IMAGE 2

Cerebral calcifications in congenital toxoplasmosis are usually bilateral, measure up to 2 cm each, and may be associated with hydrocephalus. *Courtesy: Duke Duncan.*

Trachoma

EPIDEMIOLOGY

Trachoma is caused by the obligate intracellular bacterium *Chlamydia trachomatis* and is the leading cause of preventable visual impairment globally. Distribution is worldwide, and disease occurs chiefly in poor communities in the tropics. Sub-Saharan Africa and Asia, parts of the Middle East, the Americas, and the Pacific Islands are most affected. Areas without clean water sources, with poor hygiene, and with crowded living conditions are at highest risk. More than 50 million people are infected with trachoma and between 3 and 10 million are blind as a result of the infection.

PATHOPHYSIOLOGY

Vision loss in trachoma results from repeated ocular infections over many years. In endemic regions, most children are first infected by a year or two of life, and toddlers constitute the principal reservoir of *C trachomatis*. The organism is spread passively within a population by flies, fomites contaminated by secretions, or possibly aerosol droplets. The cycle of repetitive infections through childhood, adolescence, and adulthood causes progressive conjunctival scarring and corneal damage. During active infections, mucopurulent keratoconjunctivitis with follicular inflammation is typical. Individual episodes heal, but with repeated infections the conjunctival damage eventually results in entropion (inward turning of the eyelid) and trichiasis (continual eyelash irritation of the cornea). Scarring of the tarsal conjunctiva, chronic inflammation, ulceration, and corneal scarring define the cicatricial phase of disease. Neovascularization and the appearance of granulation tissue, or pannus, lead to corneal opacities. Complete blindness ultimately ensues, usually in the fourth or fifth decade.

CLINICAL PRESENTATION

Up to three-quarters of children with active trachoma exhibit no symptoms. Active ocular infections are characterized by tearing, pruritis, edema, and pain. Lymphoid follicles become prominent whitish, yellow, or grey elevations. Inflammatory thickening and hyperemia of the conjunctivae are common, particularly under the tarsal plate. Depending on the frequency and severity of prior

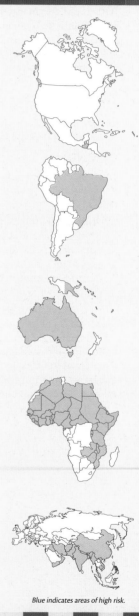

Blue indicates areas of high risk.

infections, conjunctival scarring may be present and appears as white lines or patches on an erythematous background. Herbert pits are circular depressions at the limbus (the conjunctiva-cornea junction) and are the sequelae of earlier follicles that resolved with scarring.

Following the cicatricial phase, findings consistent with chronic trachoma include neovascularization and pannus originating at the limbus and extending into the cornea. Entropion and trichiasis are often plainly visible.

DIAGNOSIS

Trachoma is diagnosed on clinical grounds when any of the following are present:

1. Five or more follicles > 0.5 mm in diameter on tarsal conjunctivae
2. Conjunctival scarring
3. Limbal follicles or Herbert pits
4. Corneal neovascularization and granulation tissue formation

During the active stage of infection, diagnosis is confirmed by demonstrating pathognomonic inclusion bodies in Giemsa-stained scrapings from tarsal follicles. Inclusion bodies appear as dark, intracellular, granular masses surrounding the epithelial cell nucleus. Fluorescein antibody stains and serologic testing are also possible.

The World Health Organization classifies trachoma into the following 5 stages:

1. Trachomatous inflammation follicular
2. Trachomatous inflammation intense
3. Trachomatous scarring of the tarsal conjunctiva
4. Trachomatous trichiasis
5. Trachomatous corneal opacity

TREATMENT AND PREVENTION

The SAFE strategy encapsulates trachoma treatment and prevention objectives: Surgery for trichiasis, Antibiotic therapy, Facial cleanliness in young children, and Environmental improvements such as latrine building and improved access to water to reduce transmission. Single-dose azithromycin is the antibiotic of choice. Annual mass treatment of populations with moderate or high disease prevalence has been recommended to cure sufficient numbers of children such that the community's bacterial reservoir is reduced. With this approach, ocular infection rates in some regions have plummeted from 10% to 0.1% in as few as several years.

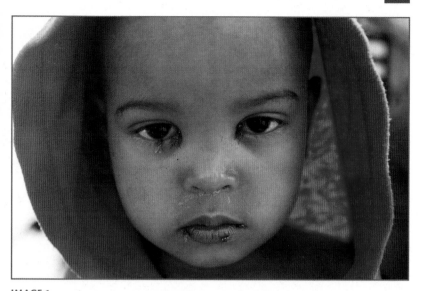

IMAGE 1
Flies are not always benign creatures. The *Musca sorbens* insect vector, which breeds in human feces, transmits trachoma. *Courtesy: Elizabeth Gilbert, International Trachoma Initiative.*

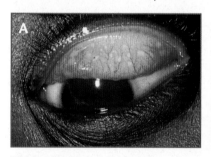
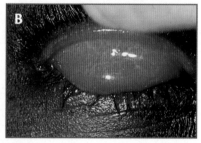

IMAGE 2A, 2B
Progressive disease is characterized here by trachomatous inflammation (Image 2A) and a papillary reaction (Image 2B). *Courtesy: Larry Schwab from* Eye Care in Developing Nations. *4th ed. London, UK: Manson Publishing Ltd; 2007.*

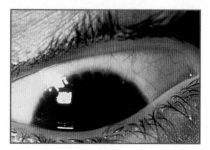

IMAGE 3
Shallow Herbert pits in the cornea follow follicle rupture and are considered to be pathognomonic for trachoma. *Courtesy: Larry Schwab from* Eye Care in Developing Nations. *4th ed. London, UK: Manson Publishing Ltd; 2007.*

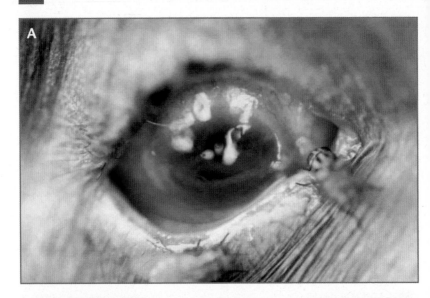

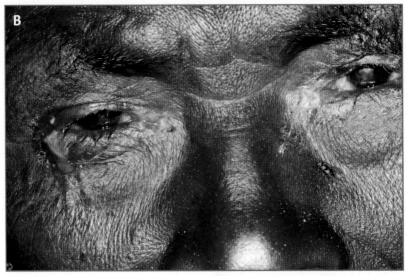

IMAGE 4A, 4B

Advanced stage trachoma (trichiasis) occurs when repeated infections scar the upper eyelid. The scars cause the lid to fold inward, making the lashes rub against the cornea with every blink, eventually leading to irreversible blindness. *Courtesy: The Carter Center.*

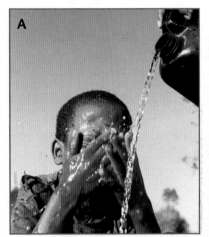 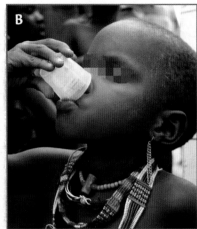

IMAGE 5A, 5B

Improved facial hygiene—even if only water is available—can prevent trachoma (Image 5A). A Sudanese girl takes a dose of banana-flavored azithromycin for protection against the bacteria that causes trachoma (Image 5B). Young children carry the highest burden of active trachoma infection and annual mass distribution of antibiotics has been recommended for communities where more than 10% of young children suffer from the disease. *Courtesy: Elizabeth Gilbert, International Trachoma Initiative (Image 5A) and The Carter Center/Paul Emerson (Image 5B).*

IMAGE 6A, 6B

World Health Organization Trachoma Grading Card. *Courtesy: World Health Organization.*

A   TRACHOMA GRADING CARD

- Each eye must be examined and assessed separately.
- Use binocular loupes (x 2.5) and adequate lighting (either daylight or a torch).
- Signs must be clearly seen in order to be considered present.

The eyelids and cornea are observed first for inturned eyelashes and any corneal opacity. The upper eyelid is then turned over (everted) to examine the conjunctiva over the stiffer part of the upper lid (tarsal conjunctiva).

The normal conjunctiva is pink, smooth, thin and transparent. Over the whole area of the tarsal conjunctiva there are normally large deep-lying blood vessels that run vertically.

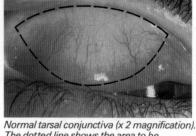

Normal tarsal conjunctiva (x 2 magnification). The dotted line shows the area to be examined.

TRACHOMATOUS INFLAMMATION – FOLLICULAR (TF): *the presence of five or more follicles in the upper tarsal conjunctiva.*

Follicles are round swellings that are paler than the surrounding conjunctiva, appearing white, grey or yellow. Follicles must be at least 0.5mm in diameter, i.e., at least as large as the dots shown below, to be considered.

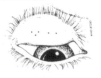

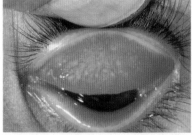

Trachomatous inflammation – follicular (TF).

TRACHOMATOUS INFLAMMATION – INTENSE (TI): *pronounced inflammatory thickening of the tarsal conjunctiva that obscures more than half of the normal deep tarsal vessels.*

The tarsal conjunctiva appears red, rough and thickened. There are usually numerous follicles, which may be partially or totally covered by the thickened conjunctiva.

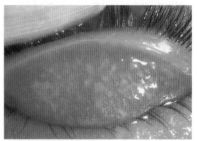

Trachomatous inflammation – follicular and intense (TF + TI).

B

TRACHOMATOUS SCARRING (TS): *the presence of scarring in the tarsal conjunctiva.*

Scars are easily visible as white lines, bands, or sheets in the tarsal conjunctiva. They are glistening and fibrous in appearance. Scarring, especially diffuse fibrosis, may obscure the tarsal blood vessels.

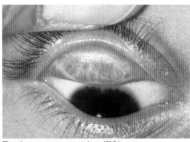
Trachomatous scarring (TS)

TRACHOMATOUS TRICHIASIS (TT): *at least one eyelash rubs on the eyeball.*

Evidence of recent removal of inturned eyelashes should also be graded as trichiasis.

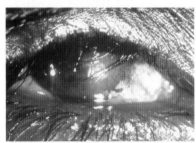
Trachomatous trichiasis (TT)

CORNEAL OPACITY (CO): *easily visible corneal opacity over the pupil.*

The pupil margin is blurred viewed through the opacity. Such corneal opacities cause significant visual impairment (less than 6/18 or 0.3 vision), and therefore visual acuity should be measured if possible.

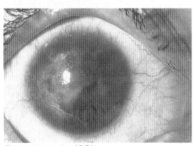
Corneal opacity (CO)

> **TF:–** give topical treatment (e.g. tetracycline 1%).
> **TI:–** give topical and consider systemic treatment.
> **TT:–** refer for eyelid surgery.

WORLD HEALTH ORGANIZATION
PREVENTION OF BLINDNESS AND DEAFNESS

Support from the partners of the WHO Alliance for the Global Elimination of Trachoma is acknowledged.

Trichuriasis

COMMON NAME

Whipworm

BACKGROUND

Trichuris trichiura is a roundworm (nematode) with a global distribution. The colloquial name is derived from the shape of adult worms, which have attenuated anterior bodies and thickened posterior ends that resemble whip handles. Whipworm is most common in the tropics, particularly in areas suffering from poor sanitation. Up to 90 % of populations can be affected in endemic regions, and approximately 800 million people, mainly children, are infected worldwide. Coinfection with other soil-transmitted helminths, including *Ascaris* and hookworm, is common.

PATHOPHYSIOLOGY

Children acquire the organism following accidental ingestion of embryonated eggs from contaminated hands or food. Eggs hatch in the small intestine and release larvae that mature to adults in the gastrointestinal lumen. Adult worms adhere to colonic mucosa by their thin anterior segments. Females, which live for a year or so, begin laying eggs several months after infection and typically produce between 3,000 and 20,000 eggs daily. Eggs passed in the stool are resilient but unembryonated and require 2 to 4 weeks of further development in soil to become infective. There is no migratory phase through the lungs, as occurs with other geohelminths.

CLINICAL PRESENTATION

Most children are asymptomatic. Heavy infections may be associated with abdominal pain, tenesmus, vomiting, constipation, and diarrhea. Frequent, bloody diarrhea characterizes *Trichuris* dysentery syndrome. Repeated tenesmus can result in intermittent or permanent rectal prolapse, which may be limited to mucosa or involve full-thickness rectal tissue. Whipworm infection can be indolent and chronic, causing colitis that mimics inflammatory bowel disease. Anemia, clubbing, and weight loss may occur. *T trichiura* has also been implicated in appendicitis.

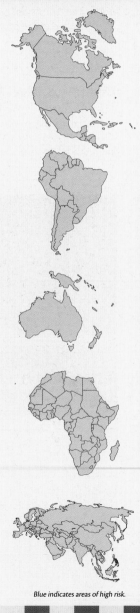

Blue indicates areas of high risk.

DIAGNOSIS

Rectal prolapse in developing world settings is commonly caused by whipworm, and worms are occasionally seen attached to the prolapsed segment. Along with direct worm visualization, definitive diagnosis can be made by identifying *T trichiura* eggs in stool.

TREATMENT AND PREVENTION

Preferred treatment is a single dose of mebendazole or albendazole. Ivermectin may also be used. Importantly, these therapies also treat other potential helminthic coinfections. Rectal prolapse generally resolves with pharmacologic treatment of worms. In severe cases, buttocks can be taped together with clean gauze sandwiched between them. Surgery is rarely necessary for prolapse repair. Attention to hand-washing and good sanitation are fundamental to preventing the fecal-oral spread of this and other soil parasites. Increasingly, mass deworming campaigns in schools are also recommended. No vaccine currently exists to prevent whipworm infection.

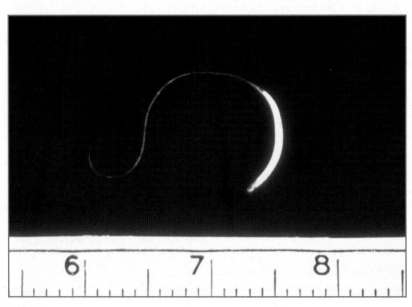

IMAGE 1

Whipworms are geohelminths, or soil-transmitted roundworms, that require no intermediate host or vector. Adult worms measure 3 to 5 cm in length. *Courtesy: Centers for Disease Control and Prevention/Mae Melvin.*

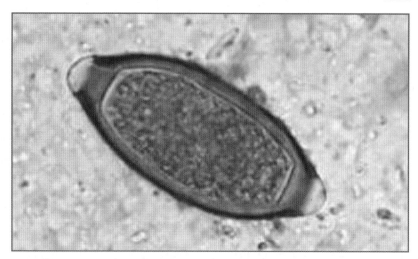

IMAGE 2

Trichuris trichiura eggs are ovoid and translucent, and have polar prominences. School-aged children who play in contaminated soil are among those with the highest exposure risk. In many poor and rural communities, transmission can take place within houses that have earth floors. *Courtesy: Centers for Disease Control and Prevention/Mae Melvin.*

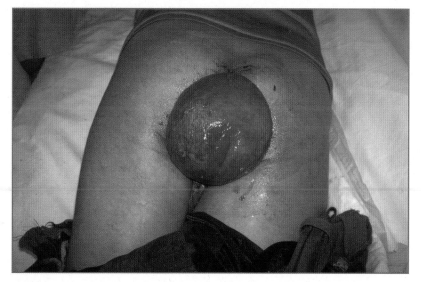

IMAGE 3

A young Guatemalan child presents with rectal prolapse. Most prolapses will spontaneously reduce. Venous stasis, edema, and ulceration can complicate those that do not. Stubborn prolapses should be reduced with gentle manual reduction using steady pressure with lubricated gloves. Buttock taping may be necessary for recurrent disease. *Courtesy: Scott Cohen.*

Trypanosomiasis, African

COMMON NAME

Sleeping sickness

BACKGROUND

African trypanosomiasis is a potentially fatal parasitic disease caused by the protozoan *Trypanosoma brucei* and transmitted by the bite of the tsetse fly. The disease is unique to tropical Africa and is endemic south of the Sahara to the Zambezi River. Two related subspecies, *T brucei gambiense* (West and Central Africa) and *T brucei rhodesiense* (East and Southern Africa), are responsible for producing generally distinct forms of clinical illness. Although it was near eradication in the 1960s, a resurgence of African trypanosomiasis has resulted from civil conflicts, population displacement, and deterioration of health systems that undermine local control initiatives. Approximately 60 million individuals in 36 African countries are at risk, and the World Health Organization (WHO) estimates that more than 300,000 people are currently infected. Threat of disease is greatest in poor, rural communities that are exposed to warm and humid environments. Peridomestic animals can acquire Gambian trypanosomiasis and may play an important epidemiological role as reservoirs of disease.

PATHOPHYSIOLOGY

Tsetse flies of genus *Glossina* ingest trypanosomes during blood meals from infected hosts. Parasites undergo morphological transformation in fly intestines and migrate to the salivary glands. Transmission occurs to naive children with subsequent bites throughout the remainder of the fly's life span, typically several months.

Following inoculation, trypanosomes travel from subcutaneous tissue through lymphatics to the bloodstream. Pathogen multiplication and dissemination define this hemolymphatic stage of infection. Circulating trypanosomes are successful at temporarily evading host immunity by altering their antigenic surface coat. Clinical disease is coincident with successive waves of parasitemia and parasite destruction. The nature of parasitemia differs in *T brucei gambiense* and *T brucei rhodesiense* infections, with the latter normally

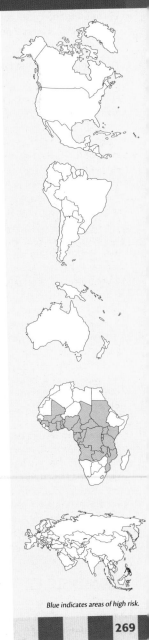

Blue indicates areas of high risk.

more virulent and continuous. In the absence of adequate treatment, parasites eventually cross the blood-brain barrier and infect the central nervous system (CNS), thereby precipitating the meningoencephalitic stage of disease.

CLINICAL PRESENTATION

The bite of the large, brown tsetse fly is a needlelike and painful insult that is often recalled by patients. Gambian trypanosomiasis comprises 90% of sleeping sickness. Incubation in this form of disease ranges from days to years (average 3 weeks). Development of a local chancre may follow inoculation. The hemolymphatic stage of infection is then associated with nonspecific fever, headache, lymphadenopathy, myalgias, arthralgias, and a pruritic rash. Winterbottom sign refers to a soft, non-tender lymphadenopathy localized to the posterior cervical chain. Central nervous system involvement (meningoencephalitic stage) appears months to years later and is characterized by sleep-wake cycle disturbances, persistent headache, confusion, and personality change. Slurred speech, focal motor weakness, tremor, and ataxia may then manifest. Late signs of illness are somnolence, seizures, coma and, ultimately, death.

Rhodesian trypanosomiasis is more aggressive. A pruritic, erythematous chancre forms at the bite site. Within weeks, infected children develop high fevers, severe headaches, chills, myalgias, and arthralgias. Symptoms are severe and acute, and progress rapidly. Death from myocarditis or multi-organ failure is possible in months, even before CNS infection.

DIAGNOSIS

The primary screening tool for Gambian trypanosomiasis is a rapid CATT (card agglutination test for trypanosomiasis) assay that tests dried blood specimens on filter paper. CATT is extremely sensitive (approaching 98%) but less specific due to cross-reactivity with animal trypanosomes, and it does not detect *T brucei rhodesiense*. The newer CIATT (card indirect agglutination test for trypanosomiasis) is an equally simple and rapid means for diagnosing both Gambian and Rhodesian trypanosomiasis but is more expensive and not widely used in endemic countries.

Demonstration of trypanosomes in blood, lymph node aspirates, or chancre aspirates is diagnostic of the hemolymphatic stage. Concentration techniques (including microhematocrit centrifugation, quantitative buffy coat, and minianion exchange column) may help to reveal organisms in cases with low-level parasitemia. Parasite detection in cerebrospinal fluid (CSF) confirms meningoencephalitic involvement; CSF pleocytosis and elevated CSF protein are supportive findings. A new Latex-IgM test for CSF trypanosomiasis is being employed more commonly.

TREATMENT AND PREVENTION

Both forms of human African trypanosomiasis are fatal without treatment. Selection of optimal pharmacologic therapy is determined by the causative subspecies and disease stage. All drugs have significant side effect profiles and should be administered with caution by experienced medical staff. Recurrences following treatment may occur. Through the recent efforts of the WHO, Médecins Sans Frontières, and pharmaceutical partners Sanofi-Aventis and Bayer AG, trypanosomiasis medications are available to endemic countries free of charge.

Hemolymphatic stage infections are treated with 7 to 10 consecutive days of intramuscular or intravenous pentamidine (for *T brucei gambiense* infection) or 6 interrupted days of intravenous suramin (for *T brucei rhodesiense* infection—treatment doses on days 1, 3, 10, 17, 24, and 31). A new oral diamidine is under clinical evaluation in several Gambian-endemic countries and may be a promising therapy for hemolymphatic stage illness.

Because treatment of CNS disease can cause considerable toxicity, lumbar puncture is necessary to confirm neurologic involvement prior to starting therapy. Meningoencephalitic disease is treated with parenteral eflornithine (for Gambian) or melarsoprol (for Gambian or Rhodesian). Eflornithine is administered 4 times daily for 2 weeks. Melarsoprol, an arsenic derivative, is particularly toxic and produces a fatal reactive encephalopathy in up to 10% of patients. Traditional dosing was 3 to 4 series of 3 to 4 injections administered every 7 to 10 days. A consecutive 10-day schedule has recently been reported to be of equivalent efficacy and is now replacing the classical regimen. Combination treatment with steroids is sometimes recommended.

Prevention and control efforts have successfully eradicated human African trypanosomiasis in many regions. Aside from active surveillance and treatment of infected individuals, public health measures focus on controlling vector populations through specially designed tsetse fly traps. Insect sterilization practices (irradiation and release of sterile male flies) exist but are expensive. Activities that reduce the likelihood of insect bites in endemic areas include use of thick clothing (flies can sting through light materials) that covers the body well and is of an unattracting neutral color.

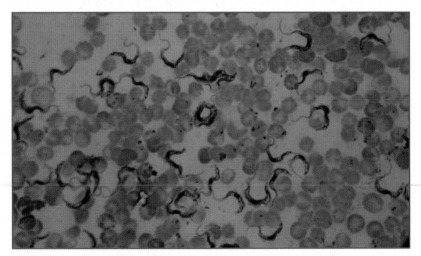

IMAGE 1

Two forms of trypanosomes are observed in human blood: stumpy and slender. Short, stumpy organisms (as seen in the center of the photograph) do not divide, but rather contribute to transmission by infecting the vector. Slender forms are metabolically highly active and multiply constantly by binary fission, with a population doubling time of 6 hours. *Trypanosoma brucei gambiense* and *Trypanosoma brucei rhodesiense* are virtually impossible to distinguish morphologically. *Courtesy: Karina Sousa and Jorge Atouguia.*

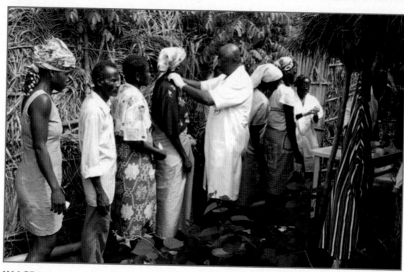

IMAGE 2

Clinical diagnosis of human African trypanosomiasis is often hampered by its intermittent course, in which asymptomatic periods are interposed with episodes of nonspecific constitutional signs and symptoms. This is particularly true for Gambian disease. Enlarged, fibrotic, non-suppurative posterior cervical lymph nodes, however, are highly sensitive for infection in endemic regions. Patients are screened for posterior cervical lymphadenopathy during active search campaigns by mobile health care teams. Patients with enlarged nodes and a positive CATT (card agglutination test for trypanosomiasis) are referred for lymph node needle aspiration. *Courtesy: Jorge Atouguia.*

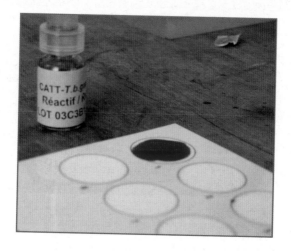

IMAGE 3

The antibody-detecting CATT (card agglutination test for trypanosomiasis) is a simple diagnostic tool that is easily performed in the field without electricity. *Courtesy: Holger Brockmeyer.*

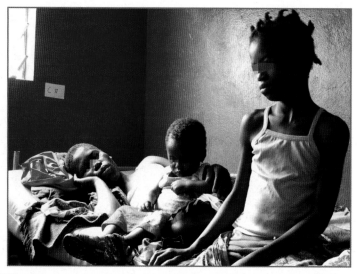

IMAGE 4

A woman is treated for meningoencephalitic Gambian trypanosomiasis in northern Angola. Treatment of late-stage disease requires intravenous drug therapy for at least 10 to 14 days. This often translates to a minimum hospital stay of nearly 3 weeks to allow for patient preparation, adverse event monitoring, and acquisition of a posttreatment cerebrospinal fluid specimen. Families frequently travel from remote villages for care. In this case, the woman had no choice but to bring her 2 children with her to the hospital. The social cost of human African trypanosomiasis is enormous. *Courtesy: Jorge Seixas and Jorge Atouguia.*

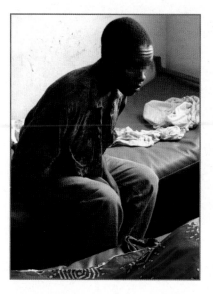

IMAGE 5

Neurologic and psychological disorders occur during meningoencephalitic human African trypanosomiasis. Unusual behaviors and mood changes are common in children. The colloquial term *sleeping sickness* stems from associated diurnal somnolence, a profound disruption of the circadian rhythm and sleep-wake cycle. *Courtesy: Holger Brockmeyer.*

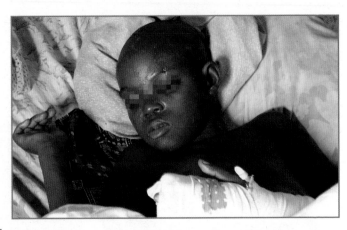

IMAGE 6

A boy suffers from severe second-stage human African trypanosomiasis. Neurologic involvement is often insidious in onset and can delay presentation. The complex clinical picture that develops—including mental, sleep, and motor disturbances—also lacks specificity and confuses the diagnosis. This patient demonstrated lassitude, delirium, and hallucinations. He had decreased muscular strength in the lower limbs and was unable to walk due to ataxia. Abnormal involuntary movements and increased muscular tonicity were present in the upper limbs. Speech was slow and slurred. *Courtesy: Jorge Seixas and Jorge Atouguia.*

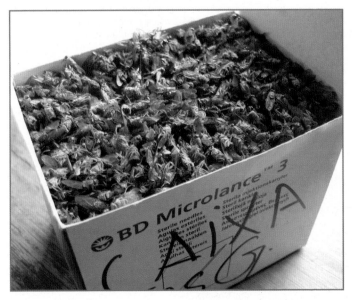

IMAGE 7

Tsetse flies are grossly similar to common houseflies but have a long proboscis that extends from the bottom of the head. This carton is filled to the brim with trapped tsetse flies. *Courtesy: Holger Brockmeyer.*

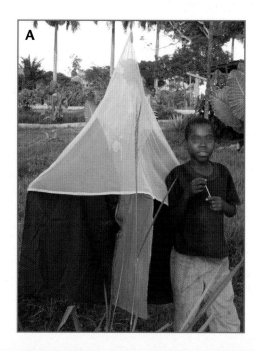

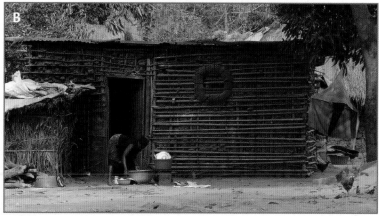

IMAGE 8A, 8B

Tsetse fly traps are the most commonly used vector control method for preventing human African trypanosomiasis in endemic regions. Blue-colored cloth attracts the insects, as do bottles filled with acetone or cow urine, which may be hung nearby. The vital importance of education in preventing disease transmission in rural communities is reflected in these images. The boy pictured next to a trap in Image 8A should not be wearing an "attractive" blue shirt. Tsetse flies are also attracted by movement; to be most effective, traps should oscillate freely in wind. The trap in Image 8B, hung against the house wall where drafts are minimal, is not optimally placed. *Courtesy: Holger Brockmeyer, Jorge Seixas, and Jorge Atouguia.*

Trypanosomiasis, American

COMMON NAME

Chagas disease

BACKGROUND

American trypanosomiasis is caused by the flagellate protozoan *Trypanosoma cruzi* and constitutes one of the most significant parasitic diseases in Central and South America. Carlos Chagas first described the pathogen in 1909 and named it for his friend and colleague Oswaldo Cruz—another Brazilian physician who was celebrated for early public health interventions targeting bubonic plague and yellow fever. In endemic countries, prevalence of Chagas disease can approach 5% of the population. Altogether, *T cruzi* is responsible for approximately 10 million current infections and more than 50,000 deaths each year.

PATHOPHYSIOLOGY

Transmission to humans is through "assassin" bugs of the family *Reduviidae* and subfamily *Triatominae*. These insects thrive in rural dwellings constructed of thatched roofs, mud walls, and adobe. Triatomines bite at night with a propensity for the mouth and eyes, hence the nickname *kissing bugs*. As the insect feeds, *T cruzi* is released in the bug's feces and then scratched or rubbed into bite wounds or facial mucosae. The conjunctivae represent a particularly common entry portal. Chagas disease can also be acquired vertically (increasing the risk of stillbirth), via blood transfusion, and by organ transplantation.

Trypomastigotes infiltrate local cells following inoculation and transform into amastigotes, which multiply intracellularly by binary fission. Parasites differentiate back to trypomastigotes, burst from cells, and disseminate hematogenously. Replication then takes place in cells all over the body, with a predilection for heart and muscle tissue. Naive triatomines take up circulating parasites during ensuing blood meals. Ingested trypomastigotes transform into epimastigotes in the vector's gastrointestinal tract, and then into infective metacyclic trypomastigotes. With subsequent biting and defecation, the cycle begins anew.

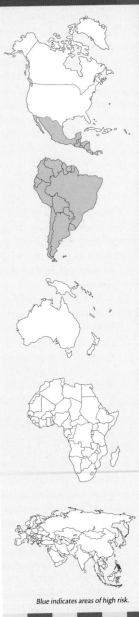

Blue indicates areas of high risk.

CLINICAL PRESENTATION

Although most individuals are asymptomatic or suffer only a nonspecific febrile illness, Chagas disease is typically characterized by 3 stages. Acute illness manifests in the first weeks following infection with fever, hepatosplenomegaly, and lymphadenopathy. This early stage corresponds to the period of active parasitemia and generally resolves spontaneously after 1 to 3 months. Romaña sign describes orbital swelling that follows conjunctival inoculation. Acute myocarditis and meningoencephalitis are rare but possible and can be life-threatening.

Second-stage disease is an intermediate phase during which children are asymptomatic. Some are thought to harbor persistent, low-level parasitemia. This stage may never progress or may slowly evolve into chronic disease.

Roughly 30% of patients suffer the chronic expression of third-stage Chagas disease, usually 1 to 2 decades after initial infection. It is unclear whether these pathologic effects result from enduring parasites, microvascular damage, or autoimmune reactions. Immunocompromised patients are more likely to progress to chronic disease. Cardiac and gastrointestinal complications are the most common and devastating. In the heart, potentially fatal rhythm abnormalities or cardiomyopathy and severe congestive heart failure occur. Histopathologically, myocardial necrosis is noted in the context of an inflammatory infiltrate. Half or more of patients with cardiac involvement acquire a left ventricular apical aneurysm. Megaesophagus or megacolon develops secondary to intramural neuron destruction and can result in incapacitating dysphagia, regurgitation, constipation, and weight loss.

DIAGNOSIS

High-level parasitemia usually develops in the early stage of infection, at which time motile trypanosomes are readily visualized by microscopic examination of fresh anticoagulated blood. Stained thick or thin blood films may also reveal parasites during this phase. Chronic infection is confirmed by biopsy or serology, though cross-reactivity with other parasitic diseases results in poor serologic specificity, and at least 2 positive tests are required to establish the diagnosis. Culture of organisms is possible with selective media, specific expertise, and time (up to 6 months). Polymerase chain reaction–based techniques exist but are primarily used in research settings. Xenodiagnosis is an indirect investigative method in which uninfected triatomines are encouraged to feed on suspected patients' blood. Insects are then sacrificed and their intestinal contents examined for metacyclic trypomastigotes. When resources permit, chronic complications may be assessed by radiologic studies (eg, abdominal radiograph and barium contrast swallow or enema) or more sophisticated cardiac and gastrointestinal evaluations (eg, electrocardiogram, Holter monitoring, echocardiography, exercise testing, and endoscopy).

TREATMENT AND PREVENTION

While it was once felt that antiparasitics were not effective beyond acute disease, it is now believed that benefits exist for treatment in all but the most advanced stages of illness, particularly in children. Nifurtimox and benznidazole are the agents used, despite their considerable side effect profile and imperfect efficacy. In early infection, treatment curbs parasitemia, shortens the symptomatic period, and can prevent long-term complications. In the intermediate period, therapy has demonstrated the ability to clear parasitemia. Some elements of chronic-stage disease may also respond to treatment, but it is likely that severe complications are irreversible. Refractory arrhythmias may necessitate medical therapy or, when feasible, pacemaker placement. Symptomatic management of congestive heart failure may be required. Medical or surgical interventions are often indicated for patients with megaesophagus or megacolon.

Vector control programs are essential for disease control in endemic countries and, fortunately, are successful. Thousands of insects can reside in a single home, and interventions at this level are especially important.

Substituting adobe with stucco cement, plastering wall cracks, and replacing thatched roofs with material such as corrugated iron are proven approaches. Dwellings at high risk can also be sprayed with pyrethroid insecticides. Insect repellent and use of mosquito bednets are important individual preventive measures. Donated blood should be screened prior to transfusion.

American trypanosomiasis is clearly a neglected disease that primarily affects people living in low-income, rural communities who are short of economic and political power. No new pharmacotherapy has been developed for the illness in more than 30 years, and no vaccine exists.

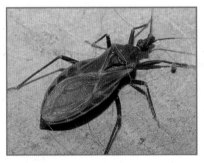

IMAGE 1

More than 130 species of triatomines exist. Most feed on vertebrate blood, and all are capable of transmitting *Trypanosoma cruzi*. Charles Darwin suffered a nighttime reduviid insect "attack" while visiting the Americas in 1835 and famously described the event in *The Voyage of the Beagle*. Fortunately for him, he evidently escaped subsequent development of chagas disease. *Courtesy: Glenn Seplak.*

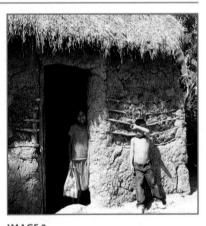

IMAGE 2

A house in Central America constructed primarily of adobe and pine needle leaves. It appears quite comfortable, but unfortunately also favors triatomine accommodation. Inside the dwellings, kissing bugs need not even fly. Many merely stumble from the structural cracks and crevices in which they live, fall to the floor or bed, and crawl onto sleeping victims. *Courtesy: J. Antonio Baeza.*

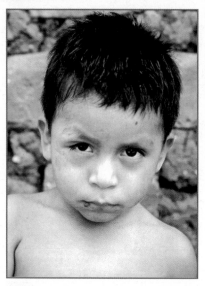

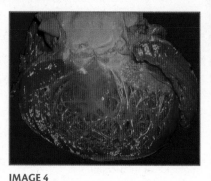

IMAGE 4

A pathologic specimen demonstrating dilated cardiomyopathy from a patient with Chagas disease in Colombia, South America. Myocarditis and conduction abnormalities are thought to be initiating events in patients with chronic trypanosomiasis-related cardiac illness. *Courtesy: María Fernanda Peña Prieto.*

IMAGE 3

A child in Panama presents with an early stage of the characteristic Romaña sign. *Courtesy: Centers for Disease Control and Prevention/Mae Melvin.*

Tuberculosis

COMMON NAME

Consumption

BACKGROUND

The World Health Organization (WHO) estimates that 2 billion people, just under a third of the world's population, are infected with *Mycobacterium tuberculosis*. This massive disease reservoir plays a substantial role in sustaining an average of 9 million new cases and 2 million tuberculosis (TB)-related deaths each year. Up to 15% of new infections occur in children, and the fractional burden of childhood illness attributed to TB can approach 40% in highly endemic regions.

PATHOPHYSIOLOGY

Transmission of *M tuberculosis* occurs primarily via inhalation of aerosolized infectious droplet nuclei that are generated from individuals with pulmonary TB. Coughing, sneezing, laughing, singing, and even speaking can expel tiny droplets that remain suspended in air for hours. Markers of close contact such as urban living, overcrowding, and lower socioeconomic status are correlated with greater risk of infection. Droplet nuclei can also be produced by cough-generating aerosol treatments, sputum induction, and lesion manipulation. Rarely, transmission occurs by direct contact with infected body fluids or fomites.

　　Following inhalation of contaminated respiratory droplets, alveolar macrophages phagocytose myco-bacteria and migrate to regional lymph nodes or other parts of the body. Subsequent interleukin production leads to activation of *M tuberculosis*–specific helper and cytotoxic T-cells. Interferon-γ is generated and enhances the ability of tissue macrophages to degrade internalized organisms, ultimately resulting in formation of characteristic granulomas. Effective cell-mediated immunity is essential for controlling infection. Children who have difficulty maintaining control of the complex immunologic relationship with invading mycobacteria are at increased risk of *M tuberculosis* disease. HIV-infected and malnourished children in particular suffer from considerably higher rates of acquisition and death from TB. The likelihood

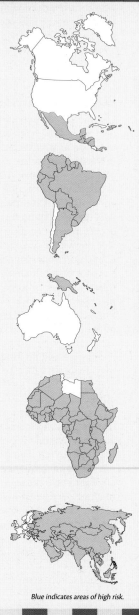

Blue indicates areas of high risk.

of progression from infection to disease is greatest shortly after initial infection and declines thereafter. Even in those who control infection initially, however, dormant mycobacteria can survive for years and reactivate later if immunity wanes. Overall, active disease develops in approximately 5% to 10% of those infected.

CLINICAL PRESENTATION

The wide spectrum of immunologic responses that children exhibit in response to *M tuberculosis* is reflected in the diverse clinical manifestations of disease that result—ranging from asymptomatic infection to hematogenous dissemination with severe or fatal disease. Pulmonary involvement occurs most frequently, but TB is also well known for causing myriad forms of extrapulmonary illness, which can be notoriously challenging to diagnose in early stages. Lymphadenitis and pleurisy are common extrapulmonary findings, followed by genitourinary, miliary (hematogenous dissemination with diffuse pulmonary lesions), bone, meningeal, and peritoneal disease. All varieties of TB occur in children, and virtually any organ system can be affected.

Constitutional symptoms include fever, night sweats, malaise, and anorexia. Wasting is common. Fever may present in varying degrees of intensity and frequency, and occasionally represents the sole expression of illness. Erythema nodosum and phlyctenular conjunctivitis are examples of type IV hypersensitivity reactions that may accompany early stage illness or appear later during disease progression.

Respiratory symptoms resulting from lung parenchymal involvement constitute a predominant clinical manifestation of TB. Chronic cough is the chief complaint, often with chest pain and production of mucopurulent sputum in older patients. Sputum may be blood-streaked, indicating that cavitation has likely occurred. Many patients are short of breath. Crepitation and wheezes may be evident on physical examination.

Non-tender lymphadenopathy, particularly of the cervical chain, can be a principal finding. External fistulization occurs in some children. Mediastinal lymph nodes, while not palpable, can be prominent in chest radiographs.

Skeletal injury can be among the most prominent of TB signs. The spinal column, hip, and knees are most frequently affected. Patients present with chronic joint pain and swelling. Vertebral involvement is associated with cord compression, kyphosis, local abscess formation, and spondylitis with gibbous deformity (ie, Pott disease). Meningitis and tuberculoma (a brain parenchymal mass) are other manifestations of central nervous system disease. Headache, irritability, fever, and vomiting may result.

Various abdominal manifestations of TB are possible. Most are painful. Esophageal and stomach ulcers lead to gastrointestinal bleeding and, in severe cases, perforation. Nonspecific diarrhea results from intestinal involvement. Peritoneal TB may cause ascites and obstruction from inflammation impinging on adjacent bowel. Mesenteric adenopathy is sometimes detectable by abdominal palpation.

Cutaneous TB (causing skin ulcers), laryngeal TB (resulting in dysphonia), and pericardial TB represent additional possible disease manifestations.

DIAGNOSIS

Latent TB is diagnosed in apparently healthy children with normal chest radiography and a positive tuberculin skin test (TST). Note, however, that the TST, while widely used, has limited diagnostic accuracy. Specificity is reduced in populations with frequent exposure to environmental mycobacteria and in those that have received bacille Calmette-Guérin (BCG) immunization. Tuberculin skin test sensitivity is particularly limited in HIV-infected, very young, and severely malnourished children.

Isolation of organisms by culture is the gold standard for diagnosis, but growth is slow and the process can be prohibitively time-consuming. Demonstrating mycobacteria in sputum smears is therefore the most commonly used method for identifying TB in adults. This technique is less useful in children owing to their limited ability to produce satisfactory sputum samples and because their sputa generally contain fewer bacilli. Microscopic examination of gastric aspirates is frequently attempted instead but may also yield false-negative results.

A number of clinical diagnostic tools have been developed to assist in the diagnosis of TB in children. Scoring systems, such as those proposed by Crofton or Edwards, assign numerical values to epidemiological and clinical features. Scores above a certain threshold predict higher likelihood of TB. While sensitivity is generally high with these tools, specificity is lower, which risks overtreatment. As such, these tools are generally recommended to serve as guides for assisting in the evaluation of children who may have TB and are not substitutes for a comprehensive assessment by an experienced health care practitioner.

No radiographic lesions are pathognomonic for TB, but chest radiographs that demonstrate parenchymal or lymph node involvement in children with risk factors is suggestive. Tissue biopsies that document typical granulomas with caseous necrosis may also be telling.

TREATMENT AND PREVENTION

Guiding principles of TB therapy are to eliminate rapidly dividing organisms, prevent relapse by eradicating one's reservoir of dormant organisms, reduce transmission, and prevent the emergence of drug resistance. Management of children with drug-susceptible pulmonary TB generally consists of 2 months of daily therapy with 4 drugs (isoniazid, rifampin, pyrazinamide, and ethambutol) followed by 4 to 7 months of treatment with 2 drugs (eg, isoniazid and rifampin). Intramuscular streptomycin is used in some regimens. Six months is currently the shortest course of therapy that is universally recommended. Fixed-dose drug combinations are available in some countries and recommended by the WHO to promote compliance. Individual treatment plans should be established in collaboration with local experts.

Most forms of extrapulmonary TB are treated with the same drugs and for a similar duration as in pulmonary disease. Tuberculous meningitis, however, may require treatment for up to 9 to 12 months. Multidrug-resistant TB (defined as resistance to isoniazid and rifampin) and extensively drug-resistant TB (resistant to isoniazid, rifampin, fluoroquinolones, and other injectable medications) require combinations of relatively poorly tolerated second-line agents for prolonged durations. Patients coinfected with *M tuberculosis* and HIV also present therapeutic challenges because many antiretroviral agents interact negatively with rifamycins.

Childhood TB usually represents primary disease transmitted from an infectious adult or adolescent and is considered to be a sentinel event in public health. In response to a new infection, local control programs should conduct a comprehensive investigation to identify the source and potential additional cases. Persons with suspected TB should be evaluated promptly. When therapy is required, appropriate medication selection and successful completion of treatment courses are critical. Directly observed therapy is the preferred, core management strategy to ensure adherence.

Bacille Calmette-Guérin vaccines have been used in nearly 4 billion people and are still routinely administered to newborns in many countries. While it does not prevent primary pulmonary TB, BCG vaccination decreases the risk of developing severe disease including meningitis and miliary TB in early childhood.

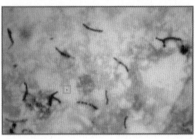

IMAGE 1

An acid-fast Ziehl-Neelsen stain reveals *Mycobacterium tuberculosis*. The organism's lipid-rich cell wall retains red carbolfuschsin stain despite washing with acid and alcohol. Bacilli are nonmotile, obligate anaerobes measuring 2 to 4 nm. Robert Koch discovered the bacterium in 1882. *Courtesy: Centers for Disease Control and Prevention/George P. Kubica.*

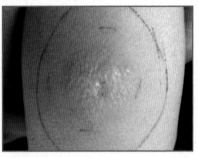

IMAGE 2

The tuberculin skin test, also known as the Mantoux test, is performed by intradermal injection of 5 U (0.1 mL) of purified protein derivative and assessing the extent of induration that develops 48 to 72 hours later. Erythema in the absence of induration is not measured. Diameter thresholds that define a positive test are determined by specific clinical and epidemiological risk factors and range from 5 to 15 mm. Induration greater than 15 mm, as seen in this child, always constitutes a positive result. *Courtesy: Leila Srour and Bryan Watt.*

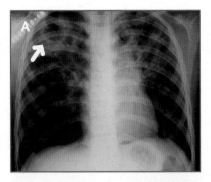

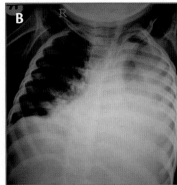

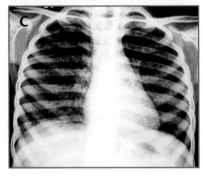

IMAGE 3A–3C

A cavitary pulmonary lesion is evident by radiography in a preadolescent Latin American girl (Image 3A). Tuberculosis (TB) can also cause pleural effusions (Image 3B). Widespread distribution of tiny lesions throughout the lungs with hematogenous dissemination describes miliary TB (Image 3C). Ghon focus is a well-circumscribed, granulomatous manifestation of primary TB infection. Its formation is usually subclinical and it tends to appear at the upper part of the lower right lobe or the lower part of the upper right lobe, where oxygen tension is high. *Courtesy: Javier Santisteban-Ponce (Image 3A) and Ashok Kapse (Image 3B, 3C).*

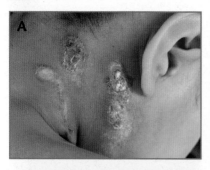

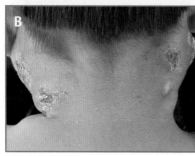

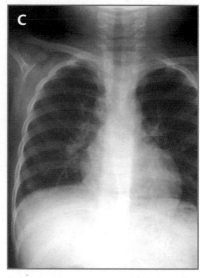

IMAGE 4A–4C

Scrofula is an old term for cervical lymphadenitis and lymphadenopathy. Most cases in children are due to non-tuberculous mycobacteria, but tuberculosis must also be considered (Image 4A, 4B). Mediastinal lymphadenopathy is a common radiographic finding in children with active disease (Image 4C). *Courtesy: Leila Srour and Bryan Watt.*

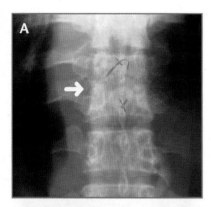

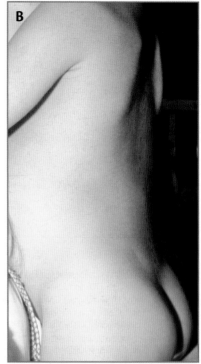

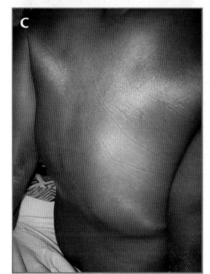

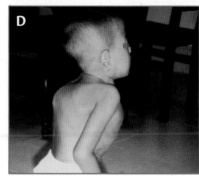

IMAGE 5A–5D

Tuberculous spondylitis leads to collapse of the vertebral bodies and destruction of intervertebral discs (Image 5A). The spectrum of clinical manifestations that results varies from flattening of normal spinal lordosis (Image 5B) to development of a severe gibbous deformity known as Pott disease (Image 5C, 5D). Spinal tuberculosis can be a devastating, disabling illness causing chronic back pain, lower extremity spasticity, and inability to walk. *Courtesy: Michael Dinerman (Image 5A), Duke Duncan (Image 5B), Phuoc V. Le (Image 5C), and Marlene Goodfriend (Image 5D).*

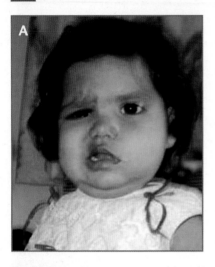
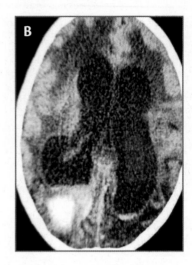

IMAGE 6A, 6B

Nervous system effects of tuberculosis (TB) take many forms. A young child in India presents with facial palsy due to TB mastoiditis (Image 6A). A 6-year-old boy in Botswana demonstrated decorticate posturing with seizures. Multiple brain tuberculomas were identified by imaging (Image 6B). The child exhibited further neurologic deterioration and died soon following the initiation of therapy. Tuberculosis is one of the most "neglected" diseases. Research and development toward diagnostic and treatment tools is grossly inadequate given the almost inconceivable global burden of disease. *Courtesy: Ashok Kapse (Image 6A) and Keri Cohn (Image 6B).*

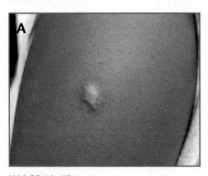
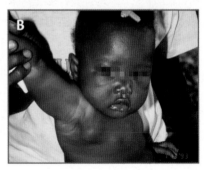

IMAGE 7A, 7B

A typical scar on the arm of an adolescent boy in the Dominican Republic marks the sign of prior bacille Calmette-Guérin (BCG) immunization (Image 7A). The vaccine is utilized in countries with high tuberculosis prevalence. Even though BCG can itself cause a positive tuberculin skin test (TST), evaluation of TST reactions in children who have received BCG are interpreted using the same criteria that are used in those who have not been vaccinated. Post-BCG regional lymphadenopathy can occur (Image 7B). Most cases resolve spontaneously, but some develop suppurative adenitis requiring surgical intervention. *Courtesy: Keri Cohn (Image 7A) and Marlene Goodfriend (Image 7B).*

Tungiasis

COMMON NAMES

Bicho de pie, Chigoe flea, Pico, Pigue

BACKGROUND

Tungiasis describes infestation of the skin with the sand flea *Tunga penetrans*. The flea inhabits warm, sandy soil in regions throughout sub-Saharan Africa and South America. The disease also occurs sporadically in Central America, the Caribbean, India, and Pakistan. Seasonal variation exists, with peak infections occurring during the dry season in the southern hemisphere. Any cutaneous surface may be affected, although in humans the flea favors the interdigital spaces, periungual and subungual areas of the toes, and the soles of the feet.

PATHOPHYSIOLOGY

T penetrans infestation evolves through 5 discrete stages, often clinically distinguished using a classification scheme called Fortaleza. In heavy infestations these stages can occur simultaneously, giving rise to a polymorphic appearance. Flea penetration (Fortaleza stage 1) begins when the gravid female burrows into the skin of its host, a process that takes between 3 to 7 hours. The head of the flea reaches the upper dermis, while the anogenital opening remains at the surface of the skin, creating an open pore through which eggs and feces are excreted onto the skin. At nearly 1 mm, *T penetrans* is the smallest known flea, and hence initial penetration of the flea into the skin is typically unnoticed.

Once embedded, the abdominal segment of the flea hypertrophies over 1 to 2 days (stage 2). Pruritis leads to scratching, which can facilitate bacterial colonization of the lesion via the open pore and promote superinfection. Clinical symptoms progress as the abdomen of the flea continues to enlarge, up to 3,000 times its initial volume (stage 3).

Once the process of expelling eggs is complete (approximately 2–3 weeks), the flea begins to involute and dies in the skin (stage 4). In stage 5, the dead flea itself is expelled, with resolution of symptoms and residual scarring. The entire process emcompasses 4 to 6 weeks.

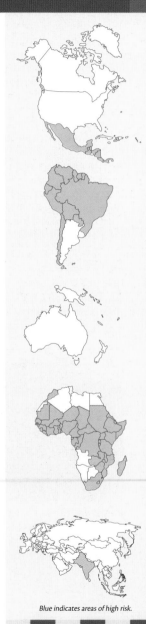

Blue indicates areas of high risk.

CLINICAL PRESENTATION

Symptoms correspond to Fortaleza stages. In stage 2 the flea is visible as a 1- to 2-mm black dot with surrounding erythema, accompanied by pain and pruritis. As the flea enlarges in stage 3, lesions become more inflamed and painful, sometimes making walking difficult in those whose feet are affected. Fleas may excrete eggs or helical threads of feces at this stage, both of which are sometimes visible on the skin. Stage 4 is characterized by hyperkeratosis, often with development of a black crust. Pain and pruritis begin to improve. Finally, in the final stage, expulsion of the dead flea leaves a circular, punched-out, non-tender depression in the skin.

DIAGNOSIS

Diagnosis is exclusively clinical in the developing world. Eggs visible during stage 3 appear as shiny white flecks and are pathognomonic. In returned travellers in whom the diagnosis is unknown, the lesion is often biopsied, and subsequent visualization of the body segments of the flea is diagnostic.

TREATMENT AND PREVENTION

Definitive treatment of tungiasis is surgical removal of fleas by unroofing lesions with a sterile instrument and debriding pore contents. Topical antibiotics should be applied to guard against superinfection, and tetanus prophylaxis is indicated for susceptible individuals. No firm recommendations exist regarding medical treatment directed at the flea itself exist, but small trials suggest that oral thiabendazole or ivermectin may be effective. Primary prevention of tungiasis is achieved by wearing closed shoes to limit the initial attachment of the parasite to the skin. Domestic animals, who also frequently harbor the flea, should be treated or removed from the home.

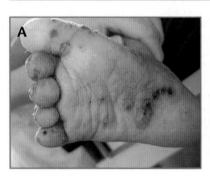 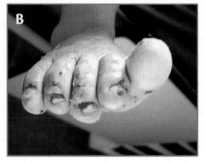

IMAGE 1A, 1B

Tunga penetrans requires a warm-blooded host to reproduce. Single lesions appear as a slowly enlarging dark-colored nodule that measures up to a centimeter in diameter. Heavy infestations can lead to severe inflammation, ulceration, and superinfection. *Courtesy: Jo Ann Gates.*

Typhoid Fever

COMMON NAME

Enteric fever

BACKGROUND

Typhoid fever is caused by *Salmonella typhi*, a gram-negative, facultative intracellular bacillus acquired by ingestion of contaminated food or water. More than 100 serotypes exist. The World Health Organization estimates that typhoid fever is responsible for 20 million infections and more than 200,000 deaths each year, primarily in underdeveloped parts of Asia, Africa, and Latin America. Incidence is as high as 500 per 100,000 people in some regions, and case-fatality rates average 1 %. *S typhi* is an increasingly virulent bacterium and multidrug-resistant strains have been identified since the 1980s. Children of all ages are at risk of disease.

Humans are the only known reservoir, and affected children harbor the organism in their bloodstream and intestinal tract. Clearance of *S typhi* generally accompanies disease resolution, but some individuals (up to 2 % of pediatric cases) continue to carry and shed the bacteria from the gallbladder following acute infection. This chronic carrier state can persist for years.

Enteric fever is a general term that encompasses illness caused by *S typhi* and *Salmonella paratyphi*, both of which are serovars of *Salmonella enterica*. Paratyphoid fever is clinically similar to typhoid fever but tends to be milder, occurs less frequently, and has a lower case-fatality rate.

PATHOPHYSIOLOGY

Typhoid fever patients and *S typhi* carriers secrete bacteria in urine and stool. Transmission takes place by accidental consumption of polluted foodstuffs. Oysters and other shellfish harvested from sewage-contaminated beds are occasional sources of infection. Once ingested, *S typhi* penetrates the epithelium of the small intestine and replicates within the reticuloendothelial cells of lymph nodes, spleen, liver, and bone marrow. Following an incubation period of 1 to 3 weeks, bacteremia ensues, and the clinical manifestations of typhoid fever develop. Release of inflammatory markers produces the fever that is almost universally observed. Bacterial shedding

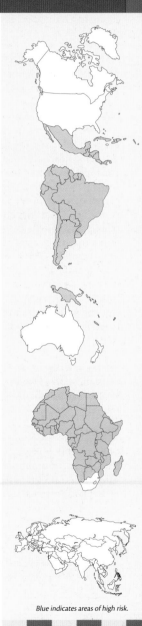

Blue indicates areas of high risk.

commonly lasts for 1 to 2 weeks after recovery. Chronic infection is defined as persistence of *S typhi* in feces for more than 6 months beyond the start of illness.

CLINICAL PRESENTATION

Clinical disease limited to diarrhea is referred to as *Salmonella gastroenteritis,* whereas *typhoid fever* denotes systemic illness. Signs and symptoms are usually non-focal. Children initially present with fever and flu-like symptoms including headache, malaise, nausea, constipation or diarrhea, and anorexia. Up to 30% of patients demonstrate the classic dermatologic finding known as *rose spots.* These blanching, maculopapular lesions usually measure 2 to 4 mm in diameter and mark the chest and abdomen. Fevers can be sustained and continue for weeks. Complications of typhoid fever include disseminated intravascular coagulation, encephalopathy, and seizures. Intestinal hemorrhage or perforation resulting from ulceration of Peyer patches in the ileum is possible and occurs in 1% of cases. Disease in infants and that caused by multidrug-resistant strains is generally more severe and is associated with higher mortality rates.

DIAGNOSIS

Children with typhoid fever often have leukopenia, thrombocytopenia, and elevated liver transaminases. The mainstay of diagnosis is blood culture. Although the yield from blood is rarely more than 60%, sensitivity can be increased when necessary by culturing bone marrow. The Widal test is a serologic assay that measures antibodies against the O and H antigens of *S typhi.* Newer serology diagnostics (eg, Typhidot and Tubex) measure specific IgM antibodies. Polymerase chain reaction (PCR), nested-PCR, and urine antigen testing are available in more sophisticated laboratories and may play a role in diagnosis in some settings.

TREATMENT AND PREVENTION

High case-fatality rates can be dramatically reduced with prompt initiation of antibiotics. Typhoid fever was traditionally treated with agents such as amoxicillin, chloramphenicol, and cotrimoxazole. However, widespread and perhaps inappropriate antibiotic use for common diarrheal illnesses is believed to have contributed to the emergence of multidrug-resistant *S typhi.* Extensive use of fluoroquinolones followed and, as expected, increasing numbers of quinolone-resistant strains have since been isolated. Cephalosporins and azithromycin remain generally effective. Awareness of local *S typhi* resistance patterns significantly improves the likelihood of administering effective therapy. Most antibiotic courses range from 7 to 14 days. Children are usually managed on an outpatient basis, but admission is required for severe cases. Fluid therapy, antipyresis, and nutrition optimization are essential treatment adjuncts.

Facilitating good sanitation and hygiene practices constitutes the best method for reducing the global burden of typhoid fever. Oral and injectable forms of vaccine against *S typhi* are available. Both are approximately 70% efficacious at 3 years' post-immunization and neither is currently approved for use in children younger than 2 years.

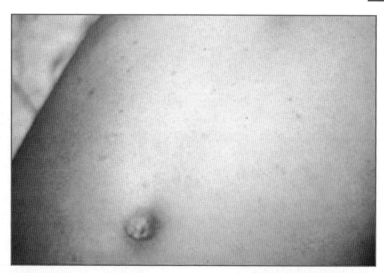

IMAGE 1

Typhoid rose spots are small, blanching, maculopapular lesions measuring 1 to 4 mm in size usually affecting the trunk. *Courtesy: C. M. Parry and Christiane Dolecek.*

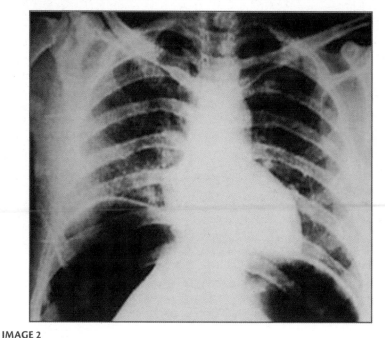

IMAGE 2

Free air under the diaphragm in a patient with suspected enteric fever is a sign of intestinal perforation, a surgical emergency. *Courtesy: Ashok Kapse.*

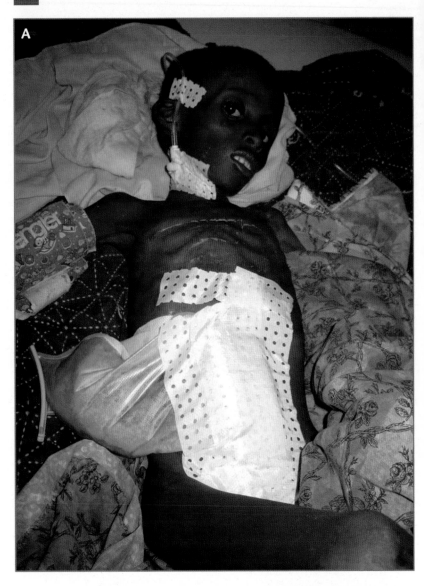

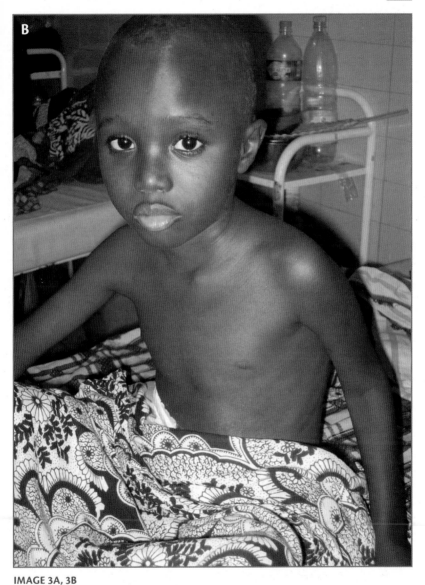

IMAGE 3A, 3B

In his third week of illness, a 10-year-old child with typhoid fever in Cote d'Ivoire developed intestinal and gallbladder perforation requiring life-saving bowel resection and ostomy placement. Following 3 months of intensive care, he was strong enough to undergo reanastomosis. *Courtesy: Keri Cohn.*

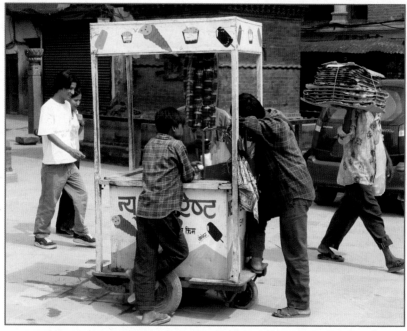

IMAGE 4

An ice cream vendor in Kathmandu, Nepal, may be selling more than tasty desserts. Ice cream is notorious for transmitting typhoid. In the late 1880s, a young Irish immigrant named Mary Mallon (known later as "Typhoid Mary") infected nearly 50 people with her popular peach ice cream. *Courtesy: Jeremy Farrar.*

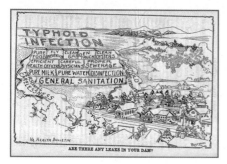

IMAGE 5

"Boil it, cook it, peel it, or forget it." Old public health messages remain remarkably current. *Courtesy: Virginia Commonwealth University Tompkins-McCaw Library.*

Varicella-Zoster and Herpes Zoster Infections

COMMON NAMES

Chickenpox, Shingles

BACKGROUND

Varicella-zoster virus (VZV), a DNA alpha-herpesvirus, is the causative agent of chickenpox and zoster. Humans are the only host. The virus is distributed worldwide but modified by geographic zones. Countries with temperate climates have a high incidence of chickenpox in children aged 5 to 9 years, and more than 90% of cases in these areas occur in the first 2 decades of life. In contrast, adults are somewhat more susceptible in tropical regions. Both sexes are equally affected.

Chickenpox season extends from end of winter to early spring. Zoster (also known as shingles) develops most commonly in adults with a history of chickenpox but can also follow varicella immunization. Zoster is not seasonal in appearance but, rather, is triggered in most cases by stress or coinfection with another virus.

PATHOPHYSIOLOGY

Primary VZV infection is transmitted by airborne spread. It is extremely contagious, and more than 80% of susceptible individuals will acquire infection if exposed to a household contact. Following inoculation at the respiratory mucosa, VZV replication occurs in regional lymph nodes and then disseminates systemically. The incubation period ranges from 10 days to 3 weeks (average 14 days). Children are contagious beginning 48 hours prior to appearance of the exanthem and remain so until all lesions have scabbed. Zoster is a late sequelae resulting from viral reactivation when cell-mediated immunity is decreased. It appears in the form of localized vesicular lesions involving the dermatomal distribution of a single or a small number of sensory nerves.

CLINICAL MANIFESTATIONS

Chickenpox is preceded in the day or two before the rash by nonspecific malaise, anorexia, headache, fever and, occasionally, abdominal pain. Cutaneous lesions begin as macules and evolve fairly rapidly to papules, vesicles, pustules, and scabs. The trunk and head are

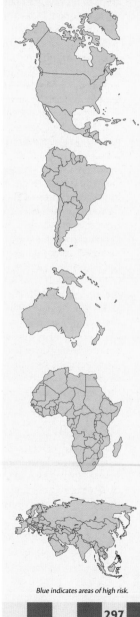

Blue indicates areas of high risk.

first involved, and then the extremities. Involvement of mucosa (mouth and conjunctiva) and scalp is possible. New crops of lesions gradually emerge over the subsequent 5 days and progressively evolve into scabs. The exanthem is characteristically polymorphic, and most non-immunized children develop up to several hundred lesions. Bacterial superinfection by *Staphylococcus aureus* or *Streptococcus pyogenes* of skin, lungs, or bone is the most frequent complication. Neurologic sequelae are rare but may consist of transient cerebellar ataxia, cerebral encephalitis, aseptic meningitis, or transverse myelitis. Varicella can be severe and even fatal in immunocompromised children, as in newborn infants who acquire varicella from their mothers in the immediate neonatal period.

Zoster seldom presents in children but may affect adolescents, particularly those with weakened immune function. A mild, unilateral vesicular skin eruption develops with minimal symptoms of acute neuritis. The dermatomal distribution is a defining feature. Lesions can become extensive. Complications include post-herpetic neuralgia, conjunctivitis, dendritic keratitis, anterior uveitis, retinitis, and facial paralysis.

DIAGNOSIS

Diagnosis of VZV infection is generally straightforward given the distinctive nature of the rash and usual history of exposure. Laboratory diagnosis is possible by serology or detection of antigens from epithelial cells at the base of newly formed vesicles.

TREATMENT AND PREVENTION

Supportive care measures include fluid management, antihistamines, antipyretics, and clipping fingernails to prevent scratch-induced excoriation. Oral acyclovir administered in the first day to otherwise healthy children with chickenpox may result in less fever, fewer days to the appearance of new lesions, and fewer lesions overall. On the other hand, prophylactic acyclovir following exposure in asymptomatic children has not been shown to be beneficial. Immunocompromised patients should be treated aggressively with intravenous acyclovir. Valacyclovir and famciclovir are potential new therapies, but experience with children is limited.

Inpatients with chickenpox must be isolated in a negative-pressure room to avoid transmission. Varicella-zoster immune globulin is indicated for exposed newborns and immunocompromised patients (eg, those with leukemia, AIDS, and transplants). Varicella vaccine, developed 30 years ago in Japan, is the most important intervention and is extremely effective in preventing severe disease. The American Academy of Pediatrics recommends immunization at 12 months of age followed by a booster at age 4. Vaccination of naive children within 72 hours of exposure has also been found to positively influence the course of disease.

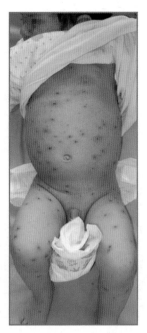

IMAGE 1

A 2-year-old immunocompetent male has classic chickenpox. Note that vesicles, papules, and scabs are present. Lesions are in different stages of development. *Courtesy: Javier Santisteban-Ponce.*

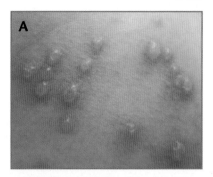

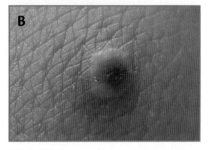

IMAGE 2A, 2B

Close inspection of individual vesicles reveals a "dewdrop on a rose petal" appearance (Image 2A). Lesions evolve to pustules and then scab (Image 2B). *Courtesy: Javier Santisteban-Ponce.*

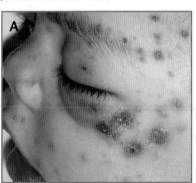

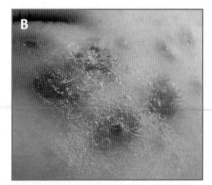

IMAGE 3A, 3B

Chickenpox in a 7-month-old infant characterized by numerous vesicles and pustules on the second day of illness (Image 3A). Eyelid edema is present, and the extent of erythema surrounding lesions is much greater than would be expected with uncomplicated varicella. A magnified view reveals yellow-brown secretions suggestive of superinfection (Image 3B). Antibiotic therapy is indicated. *Courtesy: Javier Santisteban-Ponce.*

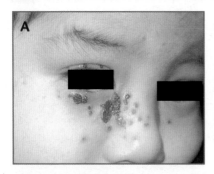

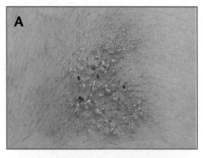

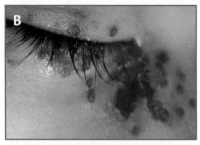

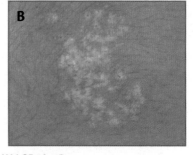

IMAGE 4A, 4B

A 2-year-old boy suffers from periorbital zoster (Image 4A). Vesicles are grouped on an erythematous base and distributed along the ophthalmic branch of the trigeminal nerve in a linear distribution. Generally, pain is minimal, and post-herpetic neuralgia is rare in children. *Courtesy: Javier Santisteban-Ponce.*

IMAGE 5A, 5B

Zoster lesions are found on the back of an 11-year-old girl who had chickenpox 5 years prior (Image 5A). A comparison is made with the same affected zone 12 days later (Image 5B). HIV serology testing should be strongly considered in children with zoster. *Courtesy: Roger Hernandez and Javier Santisteban-Ponce.*

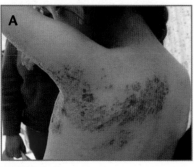

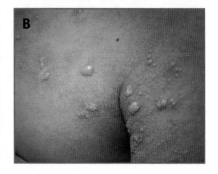

IMAGE 6A, 6B

HIV and herpes zoster in children can appear as erythematous vesicles and scabs in a dermatomal distribution (Image 6A) or vesicles and bullae with pustulous aspect and erythematous base (Image 6B). *Courtesy: Eduardo Verne.*

Viral Hemorrhagic Fever

BACKGROUND

Viral hemorrhagic fever (VHF) broadly describes a syndrome of fever, capillary leak, hemorrhage, and shock caused by enveloped RNA viruses of 4 different families: *Flavivirus* (eg, dengue, yellow fever), *Arenavirus* (eg, Lassa), *Bunyavirus* (eg, Hantavirus, Crimean-Congo, Rift Valley), and *Filovirus* (eg, Marburg, Ebola). Most of these viruses cause mild disease, but hemorrhagic forms occur and can be associated with high mortality rates.

Dengue hemorrhagic fever is transmitted by the *Aedes* day-biting mosquito and occurs worldwide in the tropics and subtropics. In most cases, it is the host's second infection with a different dengue virus strain that leads to severe forms of disease. Overall mortality rate is less than 1%.

Yellow fever also is spread by *Aedes* mosquitoes and is found in equatorial Africa and South America. Both monkeys and humans are possible reservoirs, but disease is not communicable between humans. Mortality rates range from 20% to 50%.

Lassa fever is endemic to rural West Africa and is spread through contact with certain multimammae rats or their excreta, or via body secretions of infected individuals. Mortality rates are as high as 15%. Clinically similar South American hemorrhagic fevers are caused by Junin, Machupo, Guanarito, and Whitewater Arroya viruses.

Hantavirus is found in the Far East and Europe, is spread by the excreta of rural rodents, and causes a hemorrhagic fever with renal syndrome. There is no human-to-human spread. Mortality rates are less than 15%.

Crimean-Congo hemorrhagic fever (CCHF) occurs in Africa, the Middle East, Asia, and Eastern Europe. Both domestic and wild animals can be infected, including cattle and sheep. Humans contract virus through the bite of a Hyalomma tick or through direct contact with body secretions of an infected animal or human. Mortality rates average 30%.

Rift Valley fever (RVF) is found in much of Africa and the Middle East. It is spread via mosquitoes (primarily *Aedes* and *Culicidae*) and direct contact with secretions of infected livestock. Human-to-human transmission,

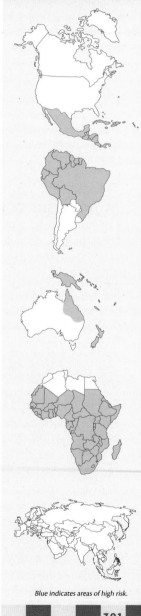

Blue indicates areas of high risk.

while not previously documented, may be possible. An associated 50% mortality rate exists.

Marburg and Ebola viruses occur in sub-Saharan Africa. Although their natural reservoirs and vectors are unknown, primates and monkeys are susceptible and transmit the infection to humans. Human-to-human spread can occur through direct skin contact, mucous membrane contact with infected body fluids, and large aerosol droplets from coughing. Household contacts, health care workers, and persons performing postmortem care are at high risk for infections. Mortality rates range from 25% to 90%.

PATHOPHYSIOLOGY

Increased capillary permeability initially manifests with edema and hemoconcentration. Effusions into serous cavities, lungs, and brain result in decreased intravascular volume, hypotension, shock, and renal failure. Direct infection of hepatocytes (particularly in yellow fever) with reactive mononuclear infiltration, fatty changes, and cellular apoptosis leads to hepatic dysfunction. Frank disseminated intravascular coagulation and death may follow.

CLINICAL PRESENTATION

Initial symptoms can mimic those of common local diseases. Index of suspicion must therefore be high to contain isolated cases and prevent nosocomial outbreaks. The incubation period varies with the etiologic virus but is generally less than 3 weeks. The list of potential manifestations is long and includes headache, myalgias, arthralgias, retrosternal chest pain, high and unremitting fever, hypothermia, petechiae or morbilliform dermatitis, frank bleeding of mucosa and skin (particularly with yellow fever, Marburg, and Ebola), conjunctival injection, icteric sclera, retinal bleeding (with RVF), sore throat with pharyngeal ulcers, bleeding gums, bloody or non-bloody vomiting and diarrhea, rectal bleeding, hepatomegaly, abdominal pain, hematuria, intractable hiccups, encephalopathy, hypotension, shock, delirium, and coma.

DIAGNOSIS

Blood smear examination may reveal rising hematocrit, leukopenia or leukocytosis, and thrombocytopenia. Hyperkalemia, hypoglycemia, acidosis, and impaired renal function may develop. Proteinuria and hematuria are possible. Elevated transaminates are universal. Coagulation abnormalities are common in most VHFs. Virus-specific serology aids with establishing diagnosis.

TREATMENT AND PREVENTION

Patient isolation is critical with VHF of unknown etiology, and public health authorities must be notified immediately. Suspected cases should be separated from confirmed cases. Isolation precautions may be relaxed if alternate diagnoses are confirmed.

Hantavirus, dengue, and yellow fever are not directly transmissible and, as such, isolation is not necessary. That said, use of mosquito nets is important for patients with dengue and yellow fever so that they are not reservoir sources for further infection. Directly transmissible VHFs include Lassa, CCHF, Marburg, Ebola and, potentially, RVF.

Supportive care is the mainstay of therapy. Fresh frozen plasma, blood transfusions, and hemodialysis may be required. Strict fluid control and intensive monitoring are essential. Cimetidine may help to reduce the risk of gastrointestinal bleeding. Ribavirin, a nucleoside analogue, is indicated early in the treatment of Lassa fever and may also be effective in CCHF, RVF, and the South American hemorrhagic fevers.

Prevention strategies vary for each virus. Cattle dipping in insecticide solution and tick repellants are used to prevent CCHF. Improved water storage practices help to guard against dengue. Individuals at high risk of contracting yellow fever should be vaccinated.

Strict barrier nursing and attention to antiseptic techniques during patient care and postmortem procedures can decrease nosocomial spread in directly transmissible VHFs. Unprotected contacts of ill patients should be quarantined for at least 3 weeks. Community education, which includes a discussion of safe burial practices, is a vital component of disease management.

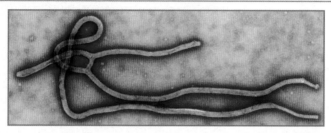

IMAGE 1

Ebola virus is named for the Ebola River in the Democratic Republic of Congo, near which the first documented outbreak occurred at a Flemish mission hospital in the mid-1970s. Morphologically, the virus is characterized by a threadlike filament measuring approximately 1,000 nm encapsulating a single RNA molecule. *Courtesy: Centers for Disease Control and Prevention/Cynthia Goldsmith.*

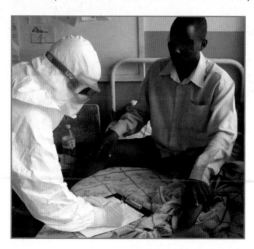

IMAGE 2

In late November 2007, the Ugandan Ministry of Health confirmed a case of Ebola in the Bundibugyo district. Many local health workers, ill-prepared to manage an Ebola outbreak, fled. Following a rapid assessment, Médecins Sans Frontières established isolation units in nearby health centers and cared for infected individuals. Community awareness and information campaigns were carried out in affected areas to reduce contamination risks, particularly during burial of disease victims. A novel Ebola virus strain was identified during this outbreak. *Courtesy: © Claude Mahoudeau/Médecins Sans Frontières.*

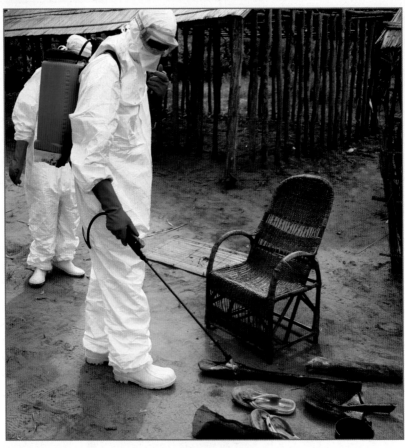

IMAGE 3

An Ebola outbreak was confirmed in West Kasai province, Democratic Republic of Congo, in September 2007. Médecins Sans Frontières treated patients and trained local health staff. The highly contagious nature of the virus means that protective material must be carefully destroyed after a single use. Contact tracing teams work toward interrupting transmission, and disinfection teams spray a strong chlorine solution over belongings at patients' homes. *Courtesy: © Pascale Zintzen/Médecins Sans Frontières.*

Vitamin A Deficiency

BACKGROUND

Vitamin A is an essential nutrient that plays important roles in vision (both nighttime and daytime), regulation of gene expression, cellular differentiation, growth and development, red blood cell production, and immune responses. The term *vitamin A* includes a broad-spectrum of related compounds such as retinol, retinol esters (retinyl palmitate), and retinoic acid. Preformed vitamin A is abundantly present in foods of animal origin and in dairy products, while vegetables and fruits are good sources of the proforms of vitamin A (also known as *carotenoids*).

Worldwide, vitamin A deficiency (VAD) is the second most prevalent nutritional disease following protein-calorie malnutrition. Vitamin A deficiency most commonly affects infants and young children, as well as pregnant and lactating women. It is estimated that worldwide 750 million people, including 140 million preschool-aged children and more than 7 million pregnant women, suffer from VAD. Globally, more than 4 million children have xerophthalmia, approximately half a million children develop blindness, and 1 to 2.5 million children die annually from VAD. Vitamin A deficiency is prevalent in tropical and subtropical regions of Africa, Asia, and the Western Pacific with almost half the cases occurring in South and Southeast Asia.

PATHOPHYSIOLOGY

The most common cause of VAD is inadequate intake Secondary VAD results from conditions associated with poor absorption, defective storage, rapid use, and excessive loss of vitamin A. Bioavailability of carotenoids depends on the manner in which food is prepared and consumed, and digestion and assimilation of vitamin A compounds are influenced by fats in the diet, bile salts, and pancreatic enzymes. More than 90% of vitamin A is stored in the liver, mostly as retinyl palmitate.

CLINICAL MANIFESTATIONS

Given the crucial role of vitamin A in the human body, VAD has wide-ranging clinical effects. Xerophthalmia is the most common clinical manifestation of VAD

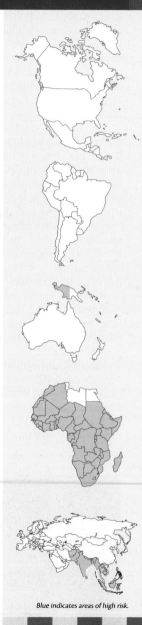

Blue indicates areas of high risk.

and a leading public health problem in the developing world. Xerophthalmia describes a spectrum of ophthalmologic disease including night blindness, conjunctival xerosis, Bitot spots, corneal xerosis, corneal ulceration, keratomalacia, corneal scars, and xerophthalmia fundus. Vitamin A deficiency disorder is the leading preventable cause of blindness among children in developing countries.

Since vitamin A is important for maintaining the integrity of epithelial tissues and for mounting cell-mediated and humoral immune responses, children with VAD have an increased frequency of respiratory infections, diarrhea, malaria, and complications from measles. In addition, HIV transmission from mother to infant occurs with greater frequency in women with VAD compared with women who have sufficient vitamin A levels.

Patients with chronic VAD typically have poor appetites and are underweight and short statured. They also have an increased tendency to develop anemia. Hyperkeratosis is a typical cutaneous manifestation of VAD, and long-standing VAD results in alopecia. Mortality from all causes among vitamin A–deficient children 6 to 72 months of age is higher than among those with normal levels.

DIAGNOSIS

The diagnosis of VAD can be definitively confirmed by measuring serum retinol levels. Serum retinol level of 40 µg/dL or higher is considered to be adequate or sufficient, 25 µg/dL to 40 µg/dL is considered marginal deficiency, 15 µg/dL to 25 µg/dL is considered to be a moderate deficiency with increased risk of mild xerophthalmia and serious infections, and less than 15 µg/dL is considered to represent severe deficiency with high risk of keratomalacia, blindness, and death.

TREATMENT AND PREVENTION

Xerophthalmia is a medical emergency. It is difficult to correct severe VAD by diet alone, and supplemental treatment with vitamin A is often required. Oral administration may be more effective than parenteral treatment.

With appropriate therapy, night blindness, corneal lesions, and Bitot spots begin resolving within days. In addition to vitamin A treatment, dietary animal and dairy products should be encouraged.

Vitamin A deficiency is highly preventable. Its incidence can be lowered by education regarding sources of vitamin A, fortification of food when necessary, and providing periodic mass supplements to at-risk populations.

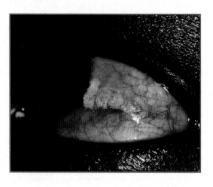

IMAGE 1

Bitot spots are an early manifestation of xerophthalmia. They result from accumulation of keratin debris and appear as foamy gray or white triangular patches in the superficial conjunctiva. *Courtesy: Larry Schwab from* Eye Care in Developing Nations. *4th ed. London, UK: Manson Publishing Ltd; 2007.*

Yaws

COMMON NAME

Frambesia tropica (tropical raspberry)

BACKGROUND

Yaws is a chronic infection caused by the spirochete *Treponema pertenue*, a subspecies of the causative agent in syphilis, *Treponema pallidum*. Transmission occurs by direct contact with infected lesions. Children who live in rural, warm, humid areas are at greatest risk, particularly where conditions of overcrowding and poor hygiene exist. Those between 6 and 10 years of age are most affected, with 75% of all cases occurring in children younger than 15 years. There is no sex or ethnic predisposition. Between 1950 and 1970, more than 50 million people were treated for yaws through a global eradication program directed by the World Health Organization (WHO) and UNICEF. Disease incidence decreased by 95% globally but, unfortunately, this dramatic public health success was not fully sustained. Yaws has reemerged since the dismantling of government programs, and renewed control efforts have been challenging due to limited resources and poor political will. While prevalence measurements are hampered by lack of consistent and accurate reporting, the WHO now estimates approximately 2.5 million people are infected worldwide. Greatest disease burdens are believed to be in parts of Southeast Asia (notably Indonesia and Timor), western Africa, and the Caribbean Islands. The extent to which the bacterium continues to cause disease in Central and South America is unclear.

PATHOPHYSIOLOGY

Although related to syphilis, yaws is not transmitted sexually. Infection results from exposure to active lesions littered with treponemes. Transmission is facilitated by breaks in recipients' skin, including those caused by insect bites. Following 9 to 90 days of incubation (average 3 weeks), an initial papilloma known as the *mother yaw*, or *frambesioma,* develops at the site of inoculation. This papular lesion, teaming with spirochetes, typically persists for up to 6 months and is responsible for seeding the body through

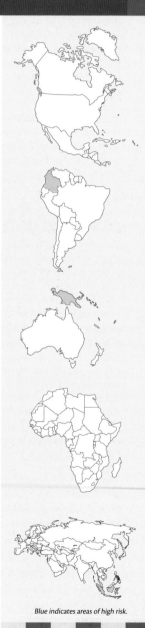

Blue indicates areas of high risk.

hematogenous, lymphatic, and local spread. Disseminated treponemes trigger a lymphocytic and plasmocytic inflammatory response in soft tissue and cartilage that leads to bouts of papules, nodules, and bone and joint swelling—usually beginning several weeks following the appearance of the mother yaw. Lesions heal spontaneously, but relapses are common. With chronic disease, inflammatory changes become irreversible. Destruction of bone, cartilage, and soft tissue occur and cause the disfiguring signs of late illness. Unlike syphilis, neurologic and cardiovascular complications are extremely rare.

CLINICAL PRESENTATION

Yaws occurs in 3 stages: early, second-stage, and late disease. Early yaws is characterized by growth of the mother yaw, a painless, skin-colored, raspberry-shaped papule at the site of initial infection. Many are pruritic, and most are found on the lower extremities. Peripheral adenopathy can be an adjunct finding. Disseminated skin lesions appear prior to or following involution of the mother yaw and herald the onset of the second disease stage. Papillomatous and hyperkeratotic growths emerge in crops and persist for months. Ulceration is possible, as are fever and dactylitis. *Crab yaws* refers to hyperkeratosis of the palms and soles that develops in some children. Early and second-stage lesions are infectious. A latency period follows, though relapses involving skin are frequent.

Late yaws develops in 10% to 20% of cases, usually 5 to 10 years after primary infection. Disfiguring erosion of skin, soft tissues, cartilage, and bone leads to monodactylitis, juxta-articular nodules, saber shins (chronic untreated osteoperiostitis of the tibia), and rhinopharyngitis mutilans (destruction of the nasal cartilage).

DIAGNOSIS

Diagnosis is chiefly by history and physical assessment. Darkfield examination of lesion biopsies in early yaws reveals spirochetes, which are 6 to 15 μm long, swarming, motile organisms. Serologic tests for syphilis, including rapid plasma reagin and Venereal Disease Research Laboratory, are positive in yaws at all stages beyond early disease. Confirmatory tests, such as fluorescent treponemal antibody absorption, are rarely required in practice.

TREATMENT AND PREVENTION

A single intramuscular injection of benzathine penicillin is curative. Tetracycline, doxycycline, or erythromycin are effective alternatives. The prognosis following treatment of early yaws is excellent, while complications of late-stage disease are irreversible. Prevention involves a 2-pronged approach: (1) improved personal hygiene and sanitation practices in endemic regions and (2) concerted efforts by local health care providers and larger government bodies to identify early yaws and provide effective therapy to curb transmission rates. Yaws is an eradicable disease. Whether resources will ever be mobilized to achieve this goal remains to be seen.

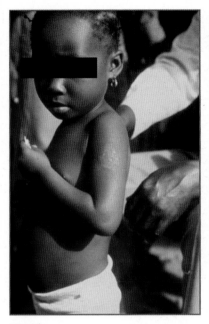

IMAGE 1
A squamous macule, seen here on the arm of a 4-year-old Ghanian girl, may be the earliest sign of yaws. This lesion has not yet matured into the primary papule that is characteristic of early stage infection. *Courtesy: Centers for Disease Control and Prevention/Peter Perine.*

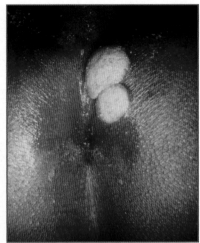

IMAGE 2
Early yaws is frequently identified by the appearance of a mother yaw (or frambesioma) at the site of inoculation. The painless, often pruritic, papilloma is highly infectious. The lesion depicted here is 1 week old. *Courtesy: Centers for Disease Control and Prevention/Peter Perine.*

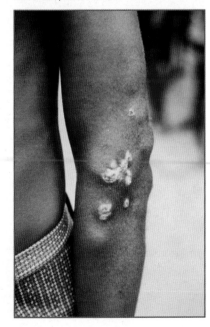

IMAGE 3
Spirochete spread from the mother yaw leads to systemic dissemination and the second stage of yaws. A child in Ghana presented with typical ulcerated nodules of 8 months' duration. *Courtesy: Centers for Disease Control and Prevention/Peter Perine.*

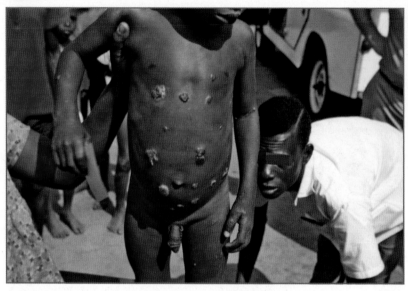

IMAGE 4

A Nigerian boy with secondary yaws. This image was captured during the late 1960s in a relief camp during the Nigerian-Biafran war. Risk of transmission is enhanced by poor environmental conditions. *Courtesy: Centers for Disease Control and Prevention/Lyle Conrad.*

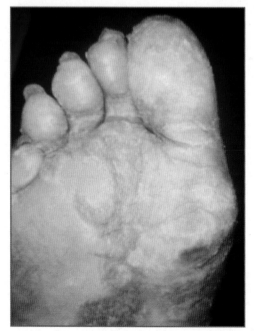

IMAGE 5

Hyperkeratotic papular lesions can develop on the soles of the feet and, less commonly, on the palms of the hands. When the soles are affected, patients may be more comfortable walking on the sides of their feet, leading to the unfortunate term *crab yaws.* *Courtesy: Centers for Disease Control and Prevention/Susan Lindsley.*

Yellow Fever

BACKGROUND

Yellow fever is caused by a flavivirus and transmitted by the *Aedes aegypti* mosquito. Disease occurs primarily in sub-Saharan Africa (90% of cases) and tropical South America. Approximately 200,000 people develop yellow fever annually, 30,000 of whom succumb to the illness. Both jungle and urban transmission cycles exist. The jungle cycle is maintained by nonhuman primates and, in Africa, is most prevalent in savanna zones during the rainy and early dry seasons. Despite the presence of the mosquito vector throughout Asia, transmission of yellow fever within Asia is not known to occur.

PATHOPHYSIOLOGY

Following inoculation the virus replicates in local lymph nodes and spreads to fixed macrophages of the liver, lung, kidneys, adrenals, spleen, and bone marrow. Hepatic histopathology overlaps with other African hemorrhagic fevers. Degenerative fatty infiltration of the myocardium and conduction system contributes to decreased cardiac output and arrhythmias. Fatty infiltration of the kidney is associated with albuminuria, tubular acidosis, and renal insufficiency. Death may result from hepatic, renal, or cardiac failure. In survivors, neutralizing antibodies lead to clearance of virus and are associated with lifelong immunity.

CLINICAL PRESENTATION

Clinical manifestations range from subclinical infection to fulminant systemic disease. Following an incubation period of 3 to 6 days, yellow fever usually manifests as a nonspecific illness characterized by mild fever and malaise. A minority of patients will have a more severe illness characterized by an abrupt onset of fever with headache, myalgias, and congestion of the conjunctivae and face. Jaundice develops shortly thereafter. The pulse may be slow relative to the elevated temperature (Faget sign), and febrile convulsions are possible, particulary in young children. Recovery generally occurs after several days but 15% to 25% of children then re-present even more acutely with fever, jaundice, vomiting, epigastric and lumbo-sacral pain, renal failure,

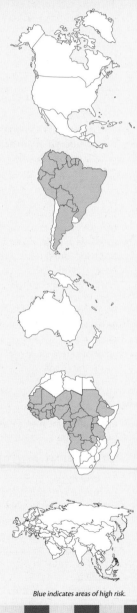

Blue indicates areas of high risk.

hemorrhagic diathesis, and an altered level of consciousness. Hypotension, shock, and metabolic acidosis may develop, worsened by myocardial dysfunction and arrhythmias. Signs of encephalopathy are common, although true encephalitis is rare. In those who recover, the convalescent phase is associated with prolonged weakness and fatigue lasting several weeks.

DIAGNOSIS

The diagnosis of yellow fever should be considered in unvaccinated children with onset of illness within a week of exposure to endemic regions of Africa or South America. The hallmark symptoms of yellow fever—jaundice and fever—are nonspecific; diagnosis must be confirmed by serology. However, in those with antecedent flavivirus infections (eg, dengue or West Nile virus), heterologous reactions may yield a false-positive result. Biochemical and hematologic abnormalities include transaminitis, hyperbilirubinemia, and leukopenia. Albuminuria is a typical feature and, when present, is evidence against other causes of viral hepatitis or hemorrhagic disease. Viral detection from blood is successful only before a humoral response develops. A liver biopsy should never be attempted because of the risk of fatal hemorrhage.

TREATMENT AND PREVENTION

Treatment is supportive. Hydration, correction of electrolyte disturbances, and management of possible hypoglycemia are essential. When available, oxygen, vasopressors, fresh frozen plasma, and vitamin K may be required. Histamine type-2 receptor antagonists and sucralfate may prevent gastric bleeding.

A highly efficacious live-attenuated vaccine against yellow fever has been available for 60 years and provides protective immunity for more than 95% of vaccine recipients. It is approved for use in children older than 9 months. Although a single dose of vaccine (0.5 mL, administered subcutaneously) may confer long-term or lifelong protection, the World Health Organization regulations mandate that travelers to endemic regions be revaccinated every 10 years. Neutralizing antibodies to yellow fever form within 7 to 10 days of vaccination.

Common adverse events to yellow fever vaccination include injection site pain or erythema, headache, malaise, and myalgia within a few days of vaccination. Since 1992, 6 cases of encephalitis and 10 cases of autoimmune neurologic disease have been reported, all in first-time vaccine recipients. Over the past 10 years, another rare adverse event associated with the vaccine, yellow fever vaccine-associated viscerotropic disease (YEL-AVD), has been detected. Formerly known as *febrile multiple organ system failure,* the clinical course is similar to naturally acquired yellow fever. The incidence of YEL-AVD is 0.3 to 0.5 cases per 100,000 doses of yellow fever vaccine administered, with the elderly most at risk. Many countries require a certificate of vaccination from travelers arriving from endemic areas; additionally some countries in Africa and 2 in South America (Bolivia and French Guiana) require an International Certificate of Vaccination from those who travel directly from the United States.

Along with vaccination, personal protection measures include applying insecticide (DEET) to exposed skin, coating clothing with permethrin, and sleeping under insecticide-treated bednets.

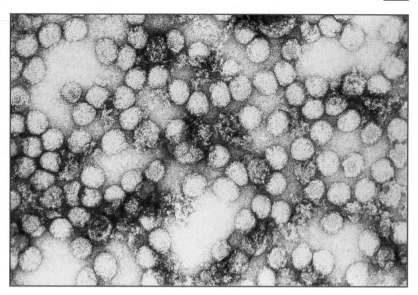

IMAGE 1

An electron micrograph depicts spheroidal yellow fever virions measuring 40 to 60 nm in diameter. Mosquito vectors acquire virus during blood meals from viremic mammals, then transmit infection to humans at subsequent feeds. The threat of epidemic transmission rises when a person with a forest-acquired infection travels to an *Aedes aegypti*–infested location while viremic. Unlike other hemorrhagic fevers, direct person-to-person transmission of yellow fever does not occur. *Courtesy: Centers for Disease Control and Prevention.*

Appendix A
Treatment Table

Topic	Drug Treatment
Ancylostomiasis	• Albendazole 400 mg PO given once, OR Mebendazole 100 mg PO given twice daily for 3 days, OR Mebendazole 500 mg PO given once, OR Pyrantel pamoate 11 mg/kg PO given once daily (max 1 g daily) for 3 days
Amebiasis	• Metronidazole 15 mg/kg PO given 3 times daily for 5–10 days, OR • Tinidazole 50 mg/kg PO given once daily (max 2 g daily) for 3 days, AND • *Follow above treatment with an intraluminal amebicide* Iodoquinol 10–12 mg/kg PO given 3 times daily (max 2 g daily) for 20 days, OR Paromomycin 10 mg/kg PO given 3 times daily for 7 days
Ascariasis	• *1–2 years of age:* albendazole 200 mg PO given once • *>2 years of age:* albendazole 400 mg PO given once, OR Mebendazole 100 mg PO given twice daily for 3 days, OR Mebendazole 500 mg PO given once, OR Pyrantel pamoate 11 mg/kg PO given once (max 1 g)
Beriberi	• Thiamine 10–25 mg IV or IM given once daily for 3 days, THEN Thiamine 10 mg PO given once daily for 2 weeks, THEN Thiamine 5 mg PO given once daily for 1 month
Buruli ulcer	• Rifampicin 10 mg/kg PO given once daily for 8 weeks, AND • Streptomycin 15 mg/kg IM given once daily for 8 weeks • Surgical debridement may be required

Topic	Drug Treatment
Carrion disease	• *Oroya Fever Stage* Ciprofloxacin 5 mg/kg IV given twice daily for 14 days, OR Chloramphenicol 12.5–25 mg/kg IV given 4 times daily PLUS Ampicillin 50 mg/kg IV given 4 times daily for 14 days • *Verruga Peruana Stage* Azithromycin 10 mg/kg PO given once daily for 7 days, OR Rifampicin 10 mg/kg PO given once daily for 14–21 days
Cholera	• Fluid resuscitation, AND • Doxycycline 100 mg PO given once
Cutaneous larva migrans	• Albendazole 400 mg PO given once daily for 3 days
Cysticercosis	• Albendazole 7.5 mg/kg PO given twice daily (max 800 mg daily) for 15–30 days, OR Praziquantel 20–30 mg/kg PO given 3 times daily for 30 days • Coadministration of corticosteroids may be recommended
Dracunculiasis	• Metronidazole 8–10 mg/kg PO given 3 times daily (max 750 mg daily) for 10 days *Not curative but may reduce inflammation.*
Giardiasis	• Metronidazole 5 mg/kg PO given 3 times daily for 5–7 days
Hydatid disease	• Albendazole 7.5 mg/kg PO given twice daily (max 800 mg daily) for 1–6 months
Hypothyroidism, congenital	• *0–6 months of age:* levothyroxine 8–10 μg/kg PO given once daily • *6–12 months of age:* levothyroxine 6–8 μg/kg PO given once daily • *1–5 years of age:* levothyroxine 5–6 μg/kg PO given once daily • *6–12 years of age:* levothyroxine 4–5 μg/kg PO given once daily

Topic	Drug Treatment
Leishmaniasis, cutaneous	• Meglumine antimoniate OR sodium stibogluconate 1–3 mL into edge of lesion and repeat if necessary • Extensive disease: either drug at 20 mg/kg IM given once daily for 30 days *Beware many possible adverse side effects with these medications.* *Must be administered under close medical supervision.*
Leishmaniasis, visceral	• Meglumine antimoniate OR sodium stibogluconate 20 mg/kg IM given once daily for 30 days • If no response: add paromomycin 15 mg/kg IM given once daily for 21 days *Beware many possible adverse side effects with these medications.* *Must be administered under close medical supervision.*
Measles	• Supportive care, AND • *6 months–1 year of age:* vitamin A 100,000 IU on days 1, 2, and 8 *>1 year of age:* vitamin A 200,000 IU on days 1, 2, and 8
Melioidosis	• Ceftazidime 30–50 mg/kg IV given 3 times daily (max 6 g daily) for 14 days, THEN • Trimethoprim-sulfamethoxazole 5 mg/kg PO given twice daily for 20 weeks, AND • Doxycycline 2 mg/kg PO given twice daily for 20 weeks, AND consider • Chloramphenicol 10 mg/kg PO given 4 times daily for 8 weeks
Meningococcemia	• Ampicillin 70 mg/kg IV given 3 times daily for 7 days, OR Ceftriaxone 50 mg/kg IV or IM given once daily for 7 days • Meningitis: ceftriaxone 100 mg/kg IV given once daily for 10–14 days

Topic	Drug Treatment
Noma	• Metronidazole 15 mg/kg IV given twice daily until improving, THEN Metronidazole 15 mg/kg PO given twice daily until afebrile, AND • Penicillin G 25,000–100,000 U/kg IV given 4 times daily until improving, THEN Penicillin VK 10–15 mg/kg PO given 3 times daily until afebrile • Consider broader spectrum antibiotics • Nutritional support
Onchocerciasis	• Ivermectin 150 µg/kg PO given once every 6–12 months until asymptomatic
Pediculosis	• Saturate wet hair with permethrin 1%, rinse after 10 minutes • Repeat application 1 week later increases efficacy • Family members may require treatment
Pellagra	• Nicotinamide 50–150 mg PO given twice daily until asymptomatic
Plague	• Streptomycin 15 mg/kg IM given twice daily for 7–10 days • Meningitis: chloramphenicol 12.5 mg/kg IV or PO given 4 times daily for 10 days • *Prophylaxis indicated for close contacts of confirmed cases.* Children: trimethoprim-sulfamethoxazole 4 mg/kg PO given twice daily for 5 days Adults: doxycycline 200 mg PO once daily for 5 days
Poststreptococcal glomerulonephritis	• *Administer if evidence of group A strep infection.* Children: penicillin VK 250 mg PO given 3 times daily for 10 days Adolescents: penicillin VK 500 mg PO given 3 times daily for 10 days
Rabies	• *Postexposure prophylaxis* Rabies vaccine 1 mL IM—5 doses given on days 0, 3, 7, 14, and 28 (administered in deltoid or anterolateral thigh muscle), AND Rabies immune globulin 20 IU/kg—half infiltrated into and around the wound, and the other half given IM at a different site than the initial rabies vaccine dose

Topic	Drug Treatment
Rickets	• Vitamin D_2 (Ergocalciferol) 2,000–5,000 IU PO given once daily for 6–12 weeks
Schistosomiasis	• *Schistosoma haematobium, S mansoni:* praziquantel 20 mg/kg given twice daily for 1 day • *S japonicum, S mekongi:* praziquantel 20 mg/kg given 3 times daily for 1 day
Scurvy	• Ascorbic acid (vitamin C) 75–150 mg PO given twice daily for 2 weeks, THEN Continue prophylactic dose 50–100 mg daily for as long as required
Syphilis	• Congenital: aqueous crystalline penicillin G 50,000 U/kg IV given twice daily for 7 days, THEN 3 times daily for 3 days • Acquired: penicillin G benzathine 50,000 U/kg IM given once (max 2.4 million U) • Neurosyphilis: aqueous crystalline penicillin G 50,000–75,000 U/kg IV given 4 times daily (max 24 million U daily) for 10–14 days
Tetanus	• *For any wounds that are not clean and minor, AND if patient's immunization cannot be confirmed* Td 0.5 mL IM (for ages 7–10) or Tdap 0.5 mL IM (for ages 11–18) given once, AND Tetanus immune globulin 3,000–6,000 U IM given once, AND Metronidazole 7.5 mg/kg PO given 4 times daily (max 4 g daily) for 10–14 days

Topic	Drug Treatment
Tinea	• *Tinea corporis, tinea cruris, tinea pedis* Topical ketoconazole once daily for 2–6 weeks, OR Topical clotrimazole twice daily for 2–6 weeks • *Tinea capitis* Microsize griseofulvin 15–20 mg/kg PO given once daily (max 1 g) for 4–6 weeks, OR Ultramicrosize griseofulvin 5–10 mg/kg PO given once daily (max 750 mg) for 4–6 weeks • *Tinea unguium* <20 kg: terbinafine 62.5 mg PO given once daily for 3 months 20–40 kg: terbinafine 125 mg PO given once daily for 3 months >40 kg: terbinafine 250 mg PO given once daily for 3 months
Toxocariasis	• Albendazole 400 mg PO given twice daily for 5 days, OR Mebendazole 100–200 mg PO given twice daily for 5 days
Toxoplasmosis	• Congenital: pyrimethamine 2 mg/kg PO given once daily for 3 days, THEN Pyrimethamine 1 mg/kg PO given once daily for 2–6 months, THEN Pyrimethamine 1 mg/kg PO given 3 times weekly for a total of 1 year, PLUS Sulfadiazine 50 mg/kg PO given twice daily for 1 year, PLUS Leucovorin 5–10 mg PO given 3 times weekly for 1 year • Acquired chorioretinitis: pyrimethamine 2 mg/kg PO given once daily (max 50 mg) for 2 days, THEN Pyrimethamine 1 mg/kg PO given once daily (max 25 mg), PLUS Sulfadiazine 50 mg/kg PO given twice daily (max 4 g daily), PLUS Leucovorin 5–20 mg PO daily, ALL until 1–2 weeks after ocular findings resolve
Trachoma	• Tetracycline 1% eye ointment to each eye twice daily for 6 weeks, OR Azithromycin 20 mg/kg PO given once (max 1 g)

Topic	Drug Treatment
Trichuriasis	• Albendazole 400 mg PO given once daily for 3 days, OR Mebendazole 100 mg PO given twice daily for 3 days, OR Mebendazole 500 mg PO given once
Trypanosomiasis, African	• *Gambiense* Hemolymphatic stage: pentamidine 4 mg/kg IM given once daily (max 300 mg) for 10 days Meningoencephalitic stage: eflornithine 100 mg/kg IV given slowly 4 times daily for 14 days • *Rhodesiense* Hemolymphatic stage: suramin 5 mg/kg IV given once daily on day 1, THEN 20 mg/kg IV once daily on days 3, 10 ,17, 24, and 31 Meningoencephalitic stage: melarsoprol 2.2 mg/kg IV given slowly once daily for 10 days *Beware many possible adverse side effects with these medications.* *May require a test dose prior to treatment.*
Trypanosomiasis, American (Chagas disease)	• *1–10 years of age:* nifurtimox 4–5 mg/kg PO given 4 times daily for 90 days *11–16 years of age:* nifurtimox 3–4 mg/kg PO given 4 times daily for 90 days, OR *1–12 years of age:* benznidazole 5 mg/kg PO given twice daily for 30–90 days
Typhoid fever	• Ciprofloxacin 15 mg/kg PO given twice daily 5–7 days, OR Ceftriaxone 75 mg/kg IV or IM given once daily for 10–14 days
Varicella	• *For severe infections, especially in those who are immunocompromised* Acyclovir 10–20 mg/kg IV given 3 times daily for 7–10 days, AND consider Varicella-zoster immune globulin 12.5 U/kg (max 625 U) given once • Neonates: acyclovir 20 mg/kg IV given 3 times daily for 14–21 days, AND consider Varicella-zoster immune globulin 125 U given once

Topic	Drug Treatment
Vitamin A deficiency	• *1–6 months of age:* vitamin A 50,000 IU PO once daily on days 1, 2, and 8 *6–11 months of age:* vitamin A 100,000 IU PO once daily on days 1, 2, and 8 *>1 year of age:* 200,000 IU PO once daily on days 1, 2, and 8
Yaws	• *1–6 years of age:* penicillin G benzathine 600,000 IU IM given once *>6 years of age:* penicillin G benzathine 1.2 million IU IM given once

Abbreviations: PO, orally; IV, intravenously; IM, intramuscularly; Td, tetanus and diphtheria toxoids; Tdap, tetanus, diphtheria, and acellular pertussis.

Appendix B
Weight-for-Height Tables

NCHS/CDC/WHO SEX COMBINED REFERENCES (1982), EXPRESSED AS PERCENTAGE OF THE MEDIAN

Length Assessed Lying Up to 84.5 cm

Length cm	Median kg	85% kg	80% kg	75% kg	70% kg	60% kg
49.0	3.2	2.7	2.6	2.4	2.3	1.92
49.5	3.3	2.8	2.6	2.5	2.3	
50.0	3.4	2.9	2.7	2.5	2.4	2.04
50.5	3.4	2.9	2.7	2.6	2.4	
51.0	3.5	3.0	2.8	2.6	2.5	2.1
51.5	3.6	3.1	2.9	2.7	2.5	
52.0	3.7	3.1	3.0	2.8	2.6	2.22
52.5	3.8	3.2	3.0	2.8	2.6	
53.0	3.9	3.3	3.1	2.9	2.7	2.34
53.5	4.0	3.4	3.2	3.0	2.8	
54.0	4.1	3.5	3.3	3.1	2.9	2.46
54.5	4.2	3.6	3.4	3.2	2.9	
55.0	4.3	3.7	3.5	3.2	3.0	2.58
55.5	4.4	3.8	3.5	3.2	3.1	
56.0	4.6	3.9	3.6	3.4	3.2	2.76
56.5	4.7	4.0	3.7	3.5	3.3	
57.0	4.8	4.1	3.8	3.6	3.4	2.88
57.5	4.9	4.2	3.9	3.7	3.4	
58.0	5.1	4.3	4.0	3.8	3.5	3.06
58.5	5.2	4.4	4.2	3.9	3.6	
59.0	5.3	4.5	4.3	4.0	3.7	3.18
59.5	5.5	4.6	4.4	4.1	3.8	
60.0	5.6	4.8	4.5	4.2	3.9	3.36
60.5	5.7	4.9	4.6	4.3	4.0	
61.0	5.9	5.0	4.7	4.4	4.1	3.54
61.5	6.0	5.1	4.8	4.5	42	
62.0	6.2	5.2	4.9	4.6	4.3	3.72
62.5	6.3	5.4	5.0	4.7	4.4	
63.0	6.5	5.5	5.2	4.8	4.5	3.9
63.5	6.6	5.6	5.3	5.0	4.6	
64.0	6.7	5.7	5.4	5.1	4.7	4.02
64.5	6.9	5.9	5.5	5.2	4.8	
65.0	7.0	6.0	5.6	5.3	4.9	4.2
65.5	7.2	6.1	5.7	5.4	5.0	
66.0	7.3	6.2	5.9	5.5	5.1	4.38

Length cm	Median kg	85% kg	80% kg	75% kg	70% kg	60% kg
66.5	7.5	6.4	6.0	5.6	5.2	
67.0	7.6	6.5	6.1	5.7	5.3	4.56
67.5	7.8	6.6	6.2	5.8	5.4	
68.0	7.9	6.7	6.3	5.9	5.5	4.74
68.5	8.0	6.8	6.4	6.0	5.6	
69.0	8.2	7.0	6.6	6.1	5.7	4.92
69.5	8.3	7.1	6.7	6.2	5.8	
70.0	8.5	7.2	6.8	6.3	5.9	5.1
70.5	8.6	7.3	6.9	6.4	6.0	
71.0	8.7	7.4	7.0	6.5	6.1	5.22
71.5	8.9	7.5	7.1	6.6	6.2	
72.0	9.0	7.6	7.2	6.7	6.3	5.4
72.5	9.1	7.7	7.3	6.8	6.4	
73.0	9.2	7.9	7.4	6.9	6.5	5.52
73.5	9.4	8.0	7.5	7.0	6.5	
74.0	9.5	8.1	7.6	7.1	6.6	5.7
74.5	9.6	8.2	7.7	7.2	6.7	
75.0	9.7	8.2	7.8	7.3	6.8	5.82
75.5	9.8	8.3	7.9	7.4	6.9	
76.0	9.9	8.4	7.9	7.4	6.9	5.94
76.5	10.0	8.5	8.0	7.5	7.0	
77.0	10.1	8.6	8.1	7.6	7.1	6.06
77.5	10.2	8.7	8.2	7.7	7.2	
78.0	10.4	8.8	8.3	7.8	7.2	6.24
78.5	10.5	8.9	8.4	7.8	7.3	
79.0	10.6	9.0	8.4	7.9	7.4	6.36
79.5	10.7	9.1	8.5	8.0	7.5	
80.0	10.8	9.1	8.6	8.1	7.5	6.48
80.5	10.9	9.2	8.7	8.1	7.6	
81.0	11.0	9.3	8.8	8.2	7.7	6.6
81.5	11.1	9.4	8.8	8.3	7.7	
82.0	11.2	9.5	8.9	8.4	7.8	6.72
82.5	11.3	9.6	9.0	8.4	7.9	
83.0	11.4	9.6	9.1	8.5	7.9	6.84
83.5	11.5	9.7	9.2	8.6	8.0	
84.0	11.5	9.8	9.2	8.7	8.1	6.9
84.5	11.6	9.9	9.3	8.7	8.2	

Height Assessed Standing From 85.0 cm

Length cm	Median kg	85% kg	80% kg	75% kg	70% kg	60% kg
85.0	12.0	10.2	9.5	9.0	8.4	7.2
85.5	12.1	10.3	9.7	9.1	8.5	7.3
86.0	12.2	10.4	9.8	9.1	8.5	7.3
86.5	12.3	10.5	9.8	9.2	8.6	7.4
87.0	12.4	10.6	9.9	9.3	8.7	7.4
87.5	12.5	10.6	10.0	9.4	8.8	7.5
88.0	12.6	10.7	10.1	9.5	8.8	7.6
88.5	12.8	10.8	10.2	9.6	8.9	7.7
89.0	12.9	10.9	10.3	9.7	9.0	7.7
89.5	13.0	11.0	10.4	9.7	9.1	7.8
90.0	13.1	11.1	10.5	9.8	9.2	7.9
90.5	13.2	11.2	10.6	9.9	9.2	7.9
91.0	13.3	11.3	10.7	10.0	9.3	8.0
91.5	13.4	11.4	10.8	10.1	9.4	8.0
92.0	13.6	11.5	10.8	10.2	9.5	8.2
92.5	13.7	11.6	10.9	10.3	9.6	8.2
93.0	13.8	11.7	11.0	10.3	9.7	8.3
93.5	13.9	11.8	11.1	10.4	9.7	8.3
94.0	14.0	11.9	11.2	10.5	9.8	8.4
94.5	14.2	12.0	11.3	10.6	9.9	8.5
95.0	14.3	12.1	11.4	10.7	10.0	8.6
95.5	14.4	12.2	11.5	10.8	10.1	8.6
96.0	14.5	12.4	11.6	10.9	10.2	8.7
96.5	14.7	12.5	11.7	11.0	10.3	8.8
97.0	14.8	12.6	11.8	11.1	10.3	8.9
97.5	14.9	12.7	11.9	11.2	10.4	8.9
98.0	15.0	12.8	12.0	11.3	10.5	9.0
98.5	15.2	12.9	12.1	11.4	10.6	9.1
99.0	15.3	13.0	12.2	11.5	10.7	9.2
99.5	15.4	13.1	12.3	11.6	10.8	9.2
100.0	15.6	13.2	12.4	11.7	10.9	9.4
100.5	15.7	13.3	12.6	11.8	11.0	9.4
101.0	15.8	13.5	12.7	11.9	11.1	9.5
101.5	16.0	13.6	12.8	12.0	11.2	9.6
102.0	16.1	13.7	12.9	12.1	11.3	9.7
102.5	16.2	13.8	13.0	12.2	11.4	9.7
103.0	16.4	13.9	13.1	12.3	11.5	9.8
103.5	16.5	14.0	13.2	12.4	11.6	9.9
104.0	16.7	14.2	13.3	12.5	11.7	10.0
104.5	16.8	14.3	13.4	12.6	11.8	10.1

Length cm	Median kg	85% kg	80% kg	75% kg	70% kg	60% kg
105.0	16.9	14.4	13.6	12.7	11.9	10.1
105.5	17.1	14.5	13.7	12.8	12.0	10.3
106.0	17.2	14.6	13.8	12.9	12.1	10.3
106.5	17.4	14.8	13.9	13.0	12.2	10.4
107.0	17.5	14.9	14.0	13.1	12.3	10.5
107.5	17.7	15.0	14.1	13.3	12.4	10.6
108.0	17.8	15.2	14.3	13.4	12.5	10.7
108.5	18.0	15.3	14.4	13.5	12.6	10.8
109.0	18.1	15.4	14.5	13.6	12.7	10.9
109.5	18.3	15.5	14.6	13.7	12.8	11.0
110.0	18.4	15.7	14.8	13.8	12.9	11.0
110.5	18.6	15.8	14.9	14.0	13.0	11.2
111.0	18.8	16.0	15.0	14.1	13.1	11.3
111.5	18.9	16.1	15.1	14.2	13.3	11.3
112.0	19.1	16.2	15.3	14.3	13.4	11.5
112.5	19.3	16.4	15.4	14.4	13.5	11.6
113.0	19.4	16.5	15.5	14.6	13.6	11.6
113.5	19.6	16.7	15.7	14.7	13.7	11.8
114.0	19.8	16.8	15.8	14.8	13.8	11.9
114.5	19.9	16.9	16.0	15.0	14.0	11.9
115.0	20.1	17.1	16.1	15.1	14.1	12.1
115.5	20.3	17.3	16.2	15.2	14.2	12.2
116.0	20.5	17.4	16.4	15.4	14.3	12.3
116.5	20.7	17.6	16.5	15.5	14.5	12.4
117.0	20.8	17.7	16.7	15.6	14.6	12.5
117.5	21.0	17.9	16.8	15.8	14.7	12.6
118.0	21.2	18.0	17.0	15.9	14.9	12.7
118.5	21.4	18.2	17.1	16.1	15.0	12.8
119.0	21.6	18.4	17.3	16.2	15.1	13.0
119.5	21.8	18.5	17.4	16.4	15.3	13.1
120.0	22.0	18.7	17.6	16.5	15.4	13.2
120.5	22.2	18.9	17.8	16.7	15.5	13.3
121.0	22.4	19.1	17.9	16.8	15.7	13.4
121.5	22.6	19.2	18.1	17.0	15.8	13.6
122.0	22.8	19.4	18.3	17.1	16.0	13.7
122.5	23.1	19.6	18.4	17.3	16.1	13.9
123.0	23.3	19.8	18.6	17.5	16.3	14.0
123.5	23.5	20.0	18.8	17.6	16.5	14.1
124.0	23.7	20.2	19.0	17.8	16.6	14.2
124.5	24.0	20.4	19.2	18.0	16.8	14.4

Length cm	Median kg	85% kg	80% kg	75% kg	70% kg	60% kg
125.0	24.2	20.6	19.4	18.2	16.9	14.5
125.5	24.4	20.8	19.6	18.3	17.1	14.6
126.0	24.7	21.0	19.7	18.5	17.3	14.8
126.5	24.9	21.2	19.9	18.7	17.5	14.9
127.0	25.2	21.4	20.1	18.9	17.6	15.1
127.5	25.4	21.6	20.4	19.1	17.8	15.2
128.0	25.7	21.8	20.6	19.3	18.0	15.4
128.5	26.0	22.1	20.8	19.5	18.2	15.6
129.0	26.2	22.3	21.0	19.7	18.4	15.7
129.5	26.5	22.5	21.2	19.9	18.6	15.9
130.0	26.8	22.8	21.4	20.1	18.7	16.0

Appendix C
Instructions for Using the Mid-Upper Arm Circumference (MUAC) Assessment

1. Taking the Measurement

MUAC should be measured on the left arm while the arm is hanging down the side of the body and is relaxed. MUAC should be measured at the mid-point between the shoulder and the tip of the elbow.

The end of the tape is fed down through the first window and up through the third window, and the measurement is read from the middle (second) window.

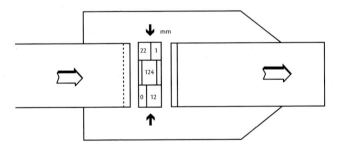

2. Reading the Measurement

MUAC can be recorded with a precision of 1 mm. Read the number in the box, which is completely visible in the middle window.

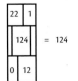

3. Interpretation

At the individual level, MUAC and weight for height are not comparable. MUAC is quick to perform, and all children can be measured with MUAC. Those children who record less than 135 mm can be referred to be measured for weight and height.

4. Interpretation With Colors

RED	=	Severely acutely malnourished
ORANGE	=	Moderately acutely malnourished
YELLOW	=	To be referred for weighing and measuring
GREEN	=	Normal

For mass screenings as long as the reading window is completely green, the children are not referred for further assessment.

Index

CHILD MID-UPPER ARM CIRCUMFERENCE MEASUREMENT

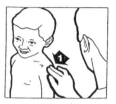

1 LOCATE TIP OF SHOULDER

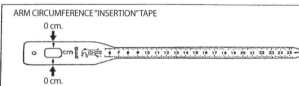

ARM CIRCUMFERENCE "INSERTION" TAPE

0 cm.

0 cm.

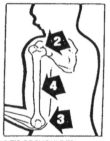

2 TIP OF SHOULDER
3 TIP OF ELBOW
4 MARK MIDPOINT

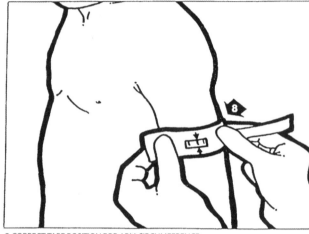

8 CORRECT TAPE POSITION FOR ARM CIRCUMFERENCE

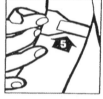

5 CORRECT TAPE TENSION

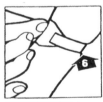

6 TAPE TOO TIGHT

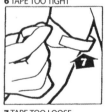

7 TAPE TOO LOOSE